Flatten my Postpartum Belly

A Simple Method to Recover from Postpartum Pooch

By Carrie Harper

Copyright

Advance Praise

"Diastasis Recti is a common condition that I often see in my practice. Carrie does a fantastic job of addressing this issue with an easy to follow approach. This book is a great resource for all women, postpartum or not, who struggle with this condition in their daily lives." – Javier Aguirre, MD, OBGYN

"Thoughtfully written, Carrie Harper explains the importance of recovery from diastasis rectus abdominus in her book Flatten My Postpartum Belly. I appreciate her emphasis on posture and daily habits as well as her steady progression of strengthening exercises. It's never too early or to late to strengthen your core - this book is for women across the span of motherhood!" - Becky Wooster, PT, DPT

Dedication

This book is dedicated to my husband, Eric, who has supported me on all of my crazy missions to help women, and to my children who inspire me to make the world a better place.

Table of Contents

Foreword

Three c-sections left my core a flabby mess that I was unable to engage. Back pain tormented me intermittently for years until a high-speed horseback-riding accident shattered any semblance of core strength I had left and sentenced me to constant, excruciating lower back pain. I saw my chiropractor three times a week. Housework put me into bed in agony. Exercise made things worse. I couldn't ride. Couldn't play. Couldn't live.

I was treating the symptoms and ignoring the root cause. I discovered Carrie's program at a point in my life when I thought I would never do the things I loved again. After the first day of breathing exercises, I felt like I'd been hit by a bus! But I stuck with the system, and within days, the back pain started to go away. With conscious effort, my core began to work again. Within six weeks, I was experiencing pain-free days. I had forgotten what pain-free felt like!

After consistently working at Carrie's program, my back pain is gone. I can ride horses and play with my kids. I don't have to plan my schedule wondering whether pain will prevent me from doing what I want to do. Carrie gave me my life back. Her program works.

Christine Stobbe, Author
www.dragonsfireseries.com

Chapter 1:

It's OK to Not Be OK

Congratulations!

Congratulations on your new baby and your new life as a Mom. I know that you are overjoyed to finally be in this stage with your baby. I know you love your role as a mother. Being a Mom is a Gift in its Truest form. Your child will teach you more about life than you ever knew possible, and your bond with baby is something that will change every aspect of your life. Parenthood teaches us a whole new level of love and affection, and it is this gift that keeps parents going, even through tough days and nights.

However.... This does not mean that life is perfect and full of rainbows. It doesn't mean that you can't wait to change diapers and you love snot bulbs. It does not mean you bounce out of bed every morning excited about every aspect of motherhood. And it does not mean that you love every colicy afternoon.

You love this baby and this life, but you might find that you are missing a piece of yourself. You might find that you don't recognize your postpartum body. You might be sad, frustrated, or upset with yourself because you look different and feel different. You also might be experiencing pain and discomfort in your abdomen, back, and pelvis. You might feel strangely weak. You might feel confused and dismayed, because this is not how you expected yourself to be postpartum. The feelings here vary, but I'm here to tell you, no matter how you are seeing yourself, your life, and your body right now, you are completely and totally normal, and there are a million other moms who feel exactly like you.

Yes, that's right. The famous woman on the cover of the magazine with the perfect abs three weeks postpartum is not real. You are real, and you are every woman. There is no shame in your joy, nor is there shame in your frustration. This is real postpartum life. These are

the things no one told you about, but should have.
Forgive them and yourself immediately, because it will
all be ok.

Stories

You may have been told something like...
"You will love EVERY second of being a mom."
"You will bounce right back to where you were before."
"You will leave the hospital in your skinny jeans."
"You will instantly get your body back and lose tons of
weight if you breastfeed."
"You will immediately embrace your new, curvy figure."
"You will be so in love with your baby that you won't
even care what you look like."

There are all kinds of reasons people tell each other
these things. Maybe that is how THEY felt. Maybe they
are hoping your experience will be better than their own.
Maybe they are trying to encourage you. Many times,
they are hiding from their own Truth, and they think that
passing on these phrases and stories will somehow help

other women embrace motherhood. But many times, these little stories that stick do a lot of emotional damage.

We as mothers and women can decide now that we will be more truthful about our own experience, and also embrace someone else's real experience as valid.

Truth

1. **Story**: "You will love EVERY second of being a mom."
   Truth: you will love being a mom! That tiny human is awesome in every possible way! However, being a new parent is exhausting, and there are a lot of things that are frustrating about this stage of life. Give yourself the grace to love yourself and your baby, but you're not required to love every *minute*.

2. **Story:** "You will bounce right back to where you were before."

   Truth: no one "bounces back." That is silly and bogus. Your body just morphed into a incubator for 9 months. Your body had to spread out to harbor another human. Your body is not a rubber band and will not bounce back. Just remember: this is not a death sentence! Every part of life is a temporary phase, and this is just one of them. Don't worry. We will help each other not bounce back, but move *forward*. Are you with me?

3. **Story:** "You will leave the hospital in your skinny jeans."

   Truth: Your hips may be wider and your abdomen may look and feel different. Many women find that their bones and joints spread while forming and carrying another human. It will take time for the hormones to change again, and for the joints and bones to change again. You may not be wearing those skinny jeans right now. Don't worry about that. Find your best sweats and rock them.

4. **Story:** "You will instantly get your body back and lose tons of weight if you breastfeed." **Truth:** Breastfeeding is great! It is nutritious for your baby and good for you. It burns about 300 calories a day (equivalent to one extra snack), which means you will not instantly burn up body fat while breastfeeding. In fact, you may feel extra hungry, and it's important to make sure to consume enough calories so that your breast milk stays optimal for baby. Instead of judging your body for any extra weight, praise your body for feeding your baby. Breastfeeding also keeps pregnancy hormones alive and well in your body, which means that your hips, pelvis, and skin may feel loose still while you're breastfeeding.

5. **Story:** "You will immediately embrace your new, curvy figure."
    Truth: you may not recognize yourself right now. You may be in total shock when you look at yourself. You may not even want to acknowledge that brave woman staring back at you. It's ok not

to embrace your lovely curves right away. This is a process. Don't be angry with yourself for not immediately embracing this change. The journey back to yourself requires taking the time to absorb this experience.

6. **Story:** "You will be so in love with your baby that you won't even care what you look like."
Truth: you will be so in love with that little person, but that does not mean that you need to forget about yourself. You are allowed to care about having strength. You are allowed to care about who you are. You are allowed to want to feel better. You are allowed to still be a person. You are the caregiver for a new life. We want you to feel fantastic about yourself. Your baby depends on your light and energy, which means that it is essential for you to care for you.

You may not feel fantastic today. You may find yourself crying a lot, confused, tired, and irritable. You might be on top of the world one minute, and then crashing the next. It's all ok. It's all postpartum life. Even if Aunt

Mildred won't admit it or has forgotten, she was there, too.

You have been incredibly focused on the life of another person, right? That life that you brought into the world is the life that you are intended to care for. And, yes, your to-do list today includes making sure that baby is safe and well-cared-for.

But what about you?

If you were that helpless being, who would you want your caregiver to be? Someone who had no sleep, didn't eat, and had no time to care for herself? Or, would you prefer a parent who was aware of her own state of health?

It's overwhelming to even consider taking care of yourself and someone else, too. I get that. We all do. But as the days turn to weeks, you will be able to find a minute for yourself again. You will sleep again. You will even be able to read again.

If you find that you are struggling with deep sadness, where you feel you cannot take care of your baby, or you are having terrible thoughts about your life or the life of your child, do not wait to take action. Depression and anxiety are common in this period of life, due to incredible shifts in hormones and lack of rest. Seek professional help immediately. If you do not have anyone to talk to, or if you can't see your doctor right away, text CONNECT to 741741. A professional will be with you right away. Don't ignore these signs of anxiety and depression:

- "Depressed mood or severe mood swings
- Excessive crying
- Difficulty bonding with your baby
- Withdrawing from family and friends
- Loss of appetite or eating much more than usual
- Inability to sleep (insomnia) or sleeping too much
- Overwhelming fatigue or loss of energy

- Reduced interest and pleasure in activities you used to enjoy
- Intense irritability and anger
- Fear that you're not a good mother
- Feelings of worthlessness, shame, guilt or inadequacy
- Diminished ability to think clearly, concentrate or make decisions
- Severe anxiety and panic attacks
- Thoughts of harming yourself or your baby
- Recurrent thoughts of death or suicide"

(source: https://www.mayoclinic.org/diseases-conditions/postpartum-depression/symptoms-causes/syc-20376617)

Your Body

By now, you recognize that your postpartum body is different from your pre-pregnancy body. Your joints and back may feel different. Your breasts may be enlarged, heavy, or uncomfortable. Your pelvis may feel wide or loose. And of course, you might be wondering what is going on in the middle of your body.

You may notice:

- I still look pregnant
- My tummy protrudes
- My navel looks weird/funny/different
- I have a lot of loose skin
- I have belly "fat"
- I have indigestion
- I have trouble with my bowels
- I have lower back pain

All of these are symptoms of Diastasis Recti, an extremely common condition for women who have ever been pregnant.

That's right. I said "ever." If you're reading this and you had your baby twenty years ago, this may still be your issue. Don't worry. We're here together today to figure out this piece of the puzzle. Together, we can change that belly situation and help you feel better. This is not just an issue of aesthetics. This is an issue of health.

Chapter 2:

My Story

I have been a fitness professional since 1994. I am an expert fitness trainer. I have taught all kinds of fitness and practices, from bootcamp to Pilates, and in 2004, I became a certified pre and post natal fitness expert.

I also got pregnant with my first child in 2004. Can you remember 2004? There was no Facebook. No Instagram. No Youtube. Mommy blogging was relatively new. There was Parenting Magazine and Babycenter.com . Those were my lifelines. I read everything, and saw that in order to have the healthiest baby, it was my job to be the healthiest mom.

Healthiest? No problem, I thought. I'm going to blow that one out of the water!

So I spent nine months eating the best foods, reading all the articles, and exercising every day. I continued teaching class, even bootcamp and Pilates. I felt GREAT. My friends marveled at my svelte physique. I was idolized by other pregnant women as I jumped around on the step at the gym, wore my gym tights, and even wore tight shirts. I was proud of my tiny frame and growing belly.

People would stop me everywhere I went, including fitness conferences, and tell me they were shocked when I turned around, because from the back, I didn't look pregnant. They considered it a compliment. I considered it a compliment. But I noticed something. When I did my abdominal work… yes, I was still doing abdominal work… my abs made a bit of a cone at the top with a squishy center. I remember telling other instructors about it, who shrugged it off and told me to be grateful my ankles weren't swelling. When I asked my ObGyn what types of fitness were ok, he said to keep doing whatever I had been doing, that I didn't have any restrictions, and that keeping my weight low was the ultimate goal.

I took my LaMaze classes like a good mommy. I knew how to breathe correctly and didn't think much of the class, but I went through the motions. I brought a magazine to class the day they showed the Cesarean video.… Because that wasn't going to be me. In fact, I had been cornered by a local man the week before who insisted that I needed to make sure I wasn't going to have a Cesarean, because way too many lazy women are having surgery to avoid doing a little work!

I hear you. It's amazing what people say to pregnant women.

My daughter tried to get here on December 20. I was having strong contractions that night and stayed awake, quietly trying to not bother anyone. The next day, I told my husband, Eric, that I thought I might be having real contractions, but that my doctor told me not to come in until they were 5 minutes apart. So I laid on the couch all day with the worst possible contractions. Contractions so bad my whole body contracted. Finally, by that afternoon, Eric had had enough of me saying no, and he took me to the hospital in our small town.

The nurses didn't fluff around; they saw I was in pain and rushed me into a room. There, we proceeded to watch Oprah and Seinfeld for hours as we waited for Jade to move along. She didn't. She was face up. Contractions were coming steadily now, and she was not moving.

Eventually, in the late-night/early morning of December 21-22, I was wheeled back to have a Cesarian. I tried desperately not to, until my doctor told me it was about to be a life threatening ordeal for Jade and myself. A few minutes and some vomit later, the doctor yelled "It's a Conehead!" as he pried my poor baby from the birth canal.

She was a Conehead, from hours of being stuck.

Jade and I stayed in the hospital for a couple of days while they carefully watched her. She had trouble keeping her body temperature up. I was struggling to move, needing more help than I thought I should. I really did not consider that I had just been through a pretty major procedure. I figured that because Cesareans are "common" that the recovery should be easy. Just a couple of hours after giving birth, the nurse pulled my catheter. I struggled for hours to go to the bathroom, until my doctor came in and saw that I needed to be recathitered. Fun.

I also remember being helped down the hallway to see my new baby through the window. I remember the nurses working overtime to help me with the baby. We finally got to spend an hour or two together as I sang Christmas carols to her in my arms. We finally came home.

She was an awful baby. I can say that now, because I have the kindest, funniest, most non-awful teenager ever. It was like she had to get it all out in the first 3 months. She didn't have a little afternoon colic; she had a 3-month-non-stop scream-fest. I thought for sure we were all going to lose our minds.

And in the midst of all of that chaos, there was me.

No longer the svelte, adorable pregnant lady, I stared at a misshapen person. She didn't even resemble me. Not only was she engorged, but there was something weird about that belly. I still looked pregnant weeks and months later. My navel looked like a pig's nose. The skin on my belly looked like the wrinkled face of Shar Pei.

I struggled to manage my household and new baby, and got angry with myself for caring about myself. I would go for days without bathing or eating, just holding a screaming baby and trying my best to soothe her.

Finally, Jade woke up one day and smiled. That was it. For her, days would now be sunny. What were long, painful days and nights were now starting to even out. She slept now and then, so I slept now and then. She and I got into a routine.

As I got into a routine, I noticed nothing was changing in my midsection. I still looked pregnant. I remember a friend looking at me and saying "what is wrong with you? What is that?" He was talking about my protruding abdomen. I was thinking the same thing.

"What IS this?" I started by asking my family. I got blank stares. "You just had a baby!" they would say. I asked friends. "Don't worry about it;" they would say, " you'll be fine. You're a trainer!" I asked members of my fitness community "You just need to strengthen your abs again, you'll be good as new!"

With my staples still in, I started doing double leg lifts. As soon as I was able, I was running with the jogger stroller. I didn't wait for anyone's clearance. I was going to be ME again!

I returned to the gym and started teaching. I hit the mats with every core move: sit ups, planks, twists, ANYTHING to get it back. Nothing worked. I felt worse with everything I tried.

I was desperately searching my periodicals and websites. There was nothing that looked like me. There was nothing that described what I was going through. There was no information about core and abdominal health postpartum. Nothing.

Finally, one day, it stared me in the face. It was a tiny sentence on the last page of Fit Pregnancy Magazine, with an asterisk. The font was around an 8, and the article had been about postpartum fitness.

*some women with extreme core weakness may have a condition called Diastasis Recti. Seek a physician's help.

Extreme core weakness? Who the heck is THAT? It's not ME. I have the strongest core of anyone I know. So I left that article and kept searching.

But something about that article bugged me. I started searching the phrase on the internet.

There was very little available, and most articles were about babies with Diastasis Recti. Finally, I found something that explained that Diastasis Recti was a condition that could happen in pregnancy, and had to do with the muscles in the core. This article, too, claimed that it was caused by muscle weakness. It took me a long time to connect those dots because these stories did not seem to apply to me, though they described my symptoms.

So, I did what anyone else would do! I asked my doctor. Keep in mind, I had seen him MANY times since I had had Jade, and he had never said a THING about my belly protruding.

"Oh, yeah!" he said, "You have the worst Diastasis I have ever SEEN!" (the man had been in medicine for like 40 years). "I'll refer you to a surgeon."

My head spun. A surgeon? The answer to my problem was a SURGEON? Oh no.

But ladies, I trusted my doctor. Right? Our doctor tells us something, and we believe it. So I believed at that moment in time, right then and there, that I had something that needed surgical correction.

This was the same doctor who told me to make no modifications to my fitness while I was pregnant and that released me to any and all forms of exercise at 8 weeks postpartum.

The surgeon told me that it would take two surgeons to correct my problem. I had a complete separation of the rectus abdominis muscle and an umbilical hernia. I believed him, too, and set up an appointment to see a plastic surgeon.

The plastic surgeon indicated that he was the answer to all I was looking for, and that when I was done having children, he and his friend would repair my abdomen. I would be as good as new.... Only BETTER, because he's that good. My life would be normal again and I could get back to the things I loved again.

Please note, it wasn't just aesthetic to me. I missed being strong in my core. I missed being able to hang from monkey bars or do somersaults or things you don't even realize are core activities. I wanted my strength back. I was desperate. And I believed him.

Years went by. We knew we wanted one more person in the family. I knew I wanted one more child, but I wasn't having a period. I went to see a chiropractor, Dr. Melissa Vrazel, who at the time was practicing in Angleton, Texas. Looking at my x-ray was quite telling. My spine had lost all of its curve. I had been trying so hard to hide my belly for so long that I had altered the muscles around my spine. Because my spine was then stick straight, every step I took was like a jackhammer into my lower back, causing not only back pain, but decreasing energy flow to my ovaries, slowing my hormones, and keeping me from having a period. On that day, I had a sudden lightbulb moment. It's All Connected.

I learned a lot from my chiropractor about posture, alignment, and how the spine and muscles work together to improve every system in the body. These are lessons I never forgot and would come in handy as I started working with other women again.

For a month, my chiropractor worked on my with spinal adjustments, acupuncture, massage, and supplements. One month later, I had a period. A month after that, I became pregnant with Cora.

Cora was a very different pregnancy. I didn't gain any extra weight, but I was terribly sickly. I had cold after cold and issue after issue. I was uncomfortable, and I knew I had no core stability holding myself together. I felt like I was falling apart. And still, I taught school (elementary music at the time), and fitness (when I could muster the strength).

Cora was delivered via planned Cesarean. She was also an awful baby, but by this time, I knew the drill. Eric and I worked in tandem with our crying, angry baby, and our adorable, happy-to-be-a-big-sister preschooler. She, like her sister, took about 3 months to get out all of her anger, and then became the happiest baby on the block, making all of our lives easier.

I took "one last shot" at healing my diastasis through someone's system that I bought online, the only system I could find in 2009. *I was a failure.* I didn't get it. I didn't understand what I was supposed to be working on, and I failed. A trainer, with all of these years of training, couldn't grasp the principles in this program. Nine weeks later, I gave up on that system and decided I would make the surgical appointment.

At the same time, my father was getting increasingly sick. My Dad had mesothelioma from working in a shipyard for a short time. My kids needed all of me, and my Dad was dying. I needed to get surgery so that I could be there for everyone, so I thought.

In June 2010, Eric drove me to Houston Methodist Hospital at something like 4 AM. On this day, I was going to be repaired by two surgeons, as we had discussed. The same day, we were expecting a phone call. My Dad would find out if there was a last treatment out there to help him, or if he was out of options.

The surgeon started marking my body with "cut here" and designs across my hips and abdomen. I started getting dizzy. This was the moment I realized that this was not a quick outpatient procedure. I looked like I was going to be cut in half in the magician's box. I was afraid. But, I shut down all of my second and third thoughts, and was wheeled down the hall for a six hour ordeal.

When I woke up, I was suffocating. I literally thought I was dying. I was gasping for air and, because I was coming out of a drug-induced stupor, I literally thought I was in a coffin. I heard someone tell me to take deep breaths. I was trying…. I couldn't breathe. I couldn't breathe! I muttered for help, and she just kept telling me to breathe.

In and out of consciousness, I heard Eric's voice. "I'm here," he said, and he sounded worried. I don't know how long it was before I was finally in my room and able to see, hear, speak, and somewhat shallow-breathe. I still didn't know why I couldn't get a breath in.

I was in that bed, propped up because I couldn't lay flat yet, when the phone rang. "How is he?" I asked my husband. "Fine," Eric said. "He's going to be fine." I knew he was lying. I could hear it in his voice, but there was nothing I could do, so I said nothing. My father was going to die.

Then came the time that I had to move. Moving my arms felt like I was pulling my chest apart. I had to use what I could to scoot to the side of my bed, and then use my hands to move my legs. It was like my legs had been completely torn off of my body. I had doll's legs.

It took my husband and a nurse to help me get to the bathroom and back. I was shocked at the fact that I felt nothing below my ribs. Nothing. Until the pain kicked in. And then, it was extreme pain, but I was still unable to move my legs.

I was in the hospital for 2 days. Two miserable soup days. I thought I was going to die every time I moved, breathed, coughed, or especially, laughed. That was dangerous being in the room with my husband, who softens every situation with humor, and who absolutely refused to leave my side. But I was finally cleared to go home, for my poor husband and in-laws to care for. I had no idea I was going to be an invalid. But there I was, In the La-Z Boy recliner, unable to do anything. My children just looked at me and had to get everything from the other adults in the house.

I was wearing a garment that hugged my abdominal wall and pelvis together, and I was not allowed to take it off. At all. Drains stuck out of my abdomen that we had to empty and clean every couple of hours. NO BATHING ALLOWED.

My husband happily took on all of it. He took care of the kids and the house, worked, and carried me to and from the hospital every day. The drains eventually came out. Still no bathing. The garment became a shorter one. Still no bathing.

It was Texas. In July. No Bathing. For 6 weeks. **SIX WEEKS**. You can imagine.

I struggled to stand up and to move. I started fighting. Every fiber of my being was wanting to stand up and fight and be myself again. And my Dad was dying. And my family needed me.

Finally, FINALLY, I was released from the doctor. No, I was not assigned a physical therapist or given any REAL further instructions. I was told to ease myself back into exercise.

How did easing myself into exercise go?
- 4 months later, I could stand up straight, with a lot of effort.
- 9 months later, I could hop.
- 1 year later, I could do a really bad, really painful sit up
- 3 years later, I could do a real sit up. One.

I became my own trainer in many ways, which I guess is how I ended up being here with you. My first self-therapy was learning how to breathe. Then to lay flat on my back. Then how to sit up, lie down, and stand up without hurting myself. Slowly, how to add strength back to not only my core, but all of me, that had been terribly weakened.

And in the midst of all of it, my father died. I was by his side, reading to him when he passed, and I stayed with my family in Virginia for a week while Jade started her first week in Kindergarten. All of it was emotionally horrible, which didn't make the physical pain any less.

Later on, in 2011 and 2012, I decided I was not going to go silently into the night of weakness and pain. I started digging into my archives of teachers and materials from the best therapeutic practices I had ever experienced: yoga and Pilates. And I went back through my notes with my chiropractor. I started really training myself, like I was training someone who had come back from any other kind of injury and surgery. I used a lot of self-talk.

- What can I feel and not feel?
- What changes when I move this part?
- How does my core feel when I do this?
- Is this movement helpful or stressful?

- Is this movement going to help me move forward or hurt me?

It was a total study of how my mind and body were reconnecting. It was an internal eye watching carefully every movement. It was a constant question "why?" I started to discover the things that were making me stronger were NOT the types of training that I had been taught in my certifications. They were NOT what I had been told by my industry.

The things that were working were the simple, small movements, the constant focus on body awareness, and the constant attention to how I was really feeling. Amazingly, I hadn't considered this before. My "before" life was very much about going heavy, hard, and strong. Now, my fit life was about restoring my mind and body together. It was about allowing myself to **FEEL**, physically, mentally, and emotionally, and that was the hardest work that I have done.

I slowly made my way back to the fitness center and back to my fit life, which was never "the same" again.

The process made me a stronger human and a better trainer. My new practices made my new fit life more efficient and more thoughtful. Little did I know that this was my calling, and that I would soon be using the same procedure to help rehabilitate many others who felt just like I once had.

Chapter 3:

Her Stories

My training process made me feel not only stronger, but actually pretty amazing. In fact, I had never felt more "together" in my life, even when I was killing it in bootcamp and doing a million sit ups. This was different. This felt like I was really strong, not just going through the motions, and that my core, all the way around, was finally functioning.

I slowly went back into training others at the gym, and this whole experience had made me curious. Was I really the ONLY one?

I started making it my practice to check every client for Diastasis Recti. Here were my statistics immediately:

- 60% of all mothers had some Diastasis

- 80% of mothers of less than one year post natal had some Diastasis
- 20% of my non-mother clients had some Diastasis

What I had found wasn't that I was alone, but that this was possibly the most under-diagnosed injury of our time.

I started using my personal system that I had developed to help myself recover from surgery, and we started journaling their Diastasis Recti and core injury recovery.

They started healing.

Client after client was reporting:
- Their bellies were flattening
- Their abdomens were getting stronger
- Their postures were getting better
- Their pain was going away
- Their digestion was getting better
- They were healing!

In 2014, I put my first 3 basic videos in a tiny course that I could distribute online. I tested it with the first 200 volunteers, and tracked them for 6 weeks. I was shocked at some of the responses that started coming back:

"I've had an injury that hasn't allowed me to workout hard. I've literally been relegated to walking. Carrie's Flat Belly System changed my life and I am so thankful to be able to work out hard again! I have many pounds to go and NOTHING is getting in my way!" -Tegan

"Been doing Carrie flat belly system for 5 weeks... I used to be soooooo self conscious of my stomach that I never took pics below my neck and always wore a jacket now I can wear shirts without hiding it anymore." -Khylah

"Super excited! I was able to go to our bootcamp class yesterday (kids with grandma, woohoo) for the first time since October when I really made my DR (diastasis recti) worse by thinking I was engaging my core but was not really doing anything with it. But thanks to Carrie's program and videos I was able to keep that mind body connection throughout the entire class. Before I went, I quickly put on her modifications video and looked at the mods for exercises I knew we were going to be doing. I went to class with the mods fresh on my mind and was practicing my breathing while driving to engage my core and somewhat signal my brain that I need to keep focused on that during the class. It was awesome!! I did the modifications and actually had to make one up on my own. And man, my lungs were on fire since I was not breathing into my stomach! Then this morning I added more reps to the supine exercises and I really feel like I'm making more of a dent. I was just following the video but this time I pushed pause after each exercise to add a few extra reps." -Faith

And on and on and on came the responses. That little document with a couple of video links ran its course for about a year. I then put together a more complete course that included everything I would teach in my training sessions. Finally, I am compiling my lessons in this book so that you can benefit from all of these therapies that I have been using to help people restore their core, get strong, heal their Diastasis Recti, and feel like themselves again.

In this book, we will explore:
- Diastasis Recti, what it is and what it means
- Diagnostics and Self-Diagnoses
- ABC's, the structure of healing
- Healing Exercises
- Life Lessons: what to do and not do
- How to Progress and Move Forward from here

I'm here to help you through the whole process. Let's begin.

Chapter 4:

Diagnosing Diastasis

Let's talk about the issues of Diastasis Recti, and let's take some time to see if this is indeed your problem. If Diastasis is NOT the issue, don't worry; the process outlined in this book can help you with all kinds of core problems and pain, not just this specific injury. Diastasis just happens to be the most prevalent abdominal injury problem, not the only one.

What is Diastasis Recti?

The underlying hammock for your entire core is called your "Transverse Abdominis." It wraps your core from front to back. On the sides are the obliques, which are muscles that help you twist. And the cover, from sternum to pelvis, down the center, is called the Rectus Abdominis.

The Rectus Abdominis is special in several ways. It is the outermost layer and easiest to see under the skin. When this muscle is developed, it has ridges in it that people call "the six pack" or "the eight pack." It is the only muscle in the body that flexes in 2 opposing directions. It can flex inward, hugging the internal organs, or it can flex outward, pushing out of the body. If you try to flex any other muscle in your body, take your biceps for example, they will only flex in one direction, even when positioned in different angles.

Another way the rectus abdominis is unique is that it has a layer of connective, mesh-like tissue holding the vertical halves together, called "linea alba." The linea alba is fluid and movable, so that the muscle can move as well.

Now, imagine the growing abdomen of a woman as she progresses in her pregnancy.

As the womb grows, the belly has to extend outward, under the abdominal walls. The transverse abdominis and the obliques usually shift and stretch for the movement, but the rectus abdominis, directly out in front of the abdomen, takes a huge strain. At some point, the rectus abdominis is likely to stretch open at the vertical center. This is when Diastasis Recti begins.

When the body begins to recover from pregnancy and the uterus shrinks, the tissue and muscle around the uterus has to take time to shift as well, and the rectus abdominis will not necessarily retain its previous shape. It is more likely to remain separated, at least temporarily, even over a year postpartum. The muscles do not necessarily close back together in the center, leaving the linea alba stretched across the abdomen. The walls of the rectus abdonimis can remain opened down the middle, anywhere along the vertical center.

Prevalence

According to research done by the Department of Sports Medicine at the Norwegian School of Sports Sciences in Norway, in a study of 300 postnatal patients, 60% had a significant Diastasis 6 weeks postpartum, and 33% still had Diastasis Recti 12 months postpartum.

In my unofficial research, working with people one on one for many years (I began checking my clients for Diastasis Recti in 2005), I have found 80% of my clients to have Diastasis Recti at 6 weeks postpartum, and if they have not undergone significant postpartum core therapy, 60% still have Diastasis Recti a year later. From there, the numbers are hard to track, but I even help women who had babies over 20 years ago with the Diastasis Recti that they either never found, or for which they never found a solution. In my practice, the numbers are staggering. Very few women are finding out that they have Diastasis Recti within that first postpartum year, and usually make assumptions about their core injury, based on what they know about physiology. They might think they have an abdominal fat problem or have loose skin around their abdomen, which may also be true, but may not be the entire issue.

I believe the reason my data is so far from the data of a medical journal is because women do not know what Diastasis Recti is, or if they do, they assume their doctor will look for it and diagnose it in their postnatal check up. In the United States of America and most countries around the world, Diastasis Recti is not part of the postnatal check up or ANY physical check up, unless the patient specifically asks to be diagnosed. At that point, the patient has usually gone through many methods, trials, and errors, in order to find something that she thinks may be the problem, but for which she does not have significant evidence. Many women never ask a doctor or therapist because they think there is no solution, because they have been told that there is no solution, or simply because they are embarrassed to ask.

Symptoms

Symptoms of Diastasis Recti Include but are not limited to:

- lower back pain
- poor posture
- constipation
- Bloating
- A bulge in the abdomen

(source: https://www.healthline.com/health/diastasis-recti#symptoms)

What Diastasis Recti Can Look Like:

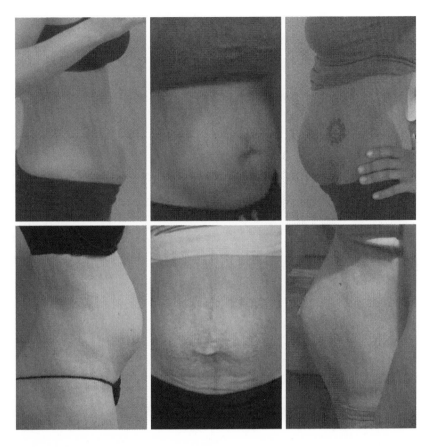

(Image Credit: anonymous clients)

Here are some images of real women with Diastasis
Recti, as seen from the outside of the skin. As you can
see, sometimes, the abdomen appears misshapen or
looks pregnant, or it looks like loose skin. That is

actually separated rectus abdominis. The separated muscle has such thin tissue holding it together that it falls forward, and can feel like it is "falling out." It can feel hard around the edges and mushy in the center. It can feel like a balloon about to pop. I have heard it described in many ways, but if your abdomen looks like one of these or feels like it is unsupported and falling out, there is a high chance it is Diastasis Recti. In the rare case, it can be extreme weakness and internal swelling, but 99% of the people I have checked with these conditions have at least some Diastasis Recti.

There are conditions other than pregnancy that can also lead to Diastasis Recti. I am seeing more and more men with this injury, usually several every day. They assume they are fat or have a "beer gut." This may be true, but their fat or swollen visceral tissue has pushed their rectus abdominis to the point of opening, and so they, too, have Diastasis Recti.

I also see Diastasis Recti in Olympic-style weight lifters. Like I previously mentioned, the rectus abdominis is the one muscle in the body that can flex inward or outward.

Heavy weight lifters sometimes press their abdominal wall outward in an attempt to support the weight they are lifting. This can cause the muscles to open. For this person, you may see an over-developed rectus abdominis that is protruding and visibly open in the middle.

Finally, I sometimes see Diastasis Recti in people who have had some kind of trauma. Some kinds of trauma include sickness, extreme weakness or illness, and eating disorders. All of these people can struggle with Diastasis Recti and assume the pain is part of the illness.

Relieving the Diastasis can also relieve the symptoms. As you can see, healing a Diastasis is not just for the aesthetics of looking good. It is to relieve pain and suffering, and to help the body. Taking care of this issue now is not a matter of vanity, but a matter of health.

Self-Diagnosis

This is a tool for self-diagnosis. Use this tool monthly to track your progress, and use it if you want to talk with a professional about your injury.

Journal your results. Keep track with pictures and measurements.

Lie on your back, like you are about to do a sit up.

- Head down
- Shoulders down
- Spine down
- Hips down
- Feet flat
- Knees bent.

Take a breath. Exhale as you curl your head and shoulders off of the floor. Get all of the air out of your abdomen, and then start your exam.

Start touching around your navel area. Do your hands sit on top of an abdominal wall, or are they going through it?

Now, move up vertically, toward your ribs, notice ridges and gaps in your abdomen there, and then work your way downward, toward the pubic bone.

BONUS MATERIAL: Follow along with me as we perform the self-check for Diastasis Recti here: https://www.youtube.com/watch?v=mQZOiqwUVQQ&t=8s

Challenges:

Sometimes, there is a lot of tissue blocking the way for your self examination. The area below the navel is sometimes the hardest part to check because that is where the transverse wraps your core. If your test is inconclusive, but you have at least one symptom from the list above, consider it some kind of core issue, in which case you are in the right place.

If you need something more conclusive, or you really want to know the details of your injury, have a physical therapist or physician check your abdomen for injury.

Check no more than once per month.

Use a cloth measuring tape for the length and width. The length is from ribs to hips, how long the injury is. The width is how many centimeters across it is at its widest point.
For the depth, use your finger tips. Can you press down to ½ of your first joint in your first finger? More than that? Can you tell that you are going all the way through the muscle?

Take notes for yourself today, to the best of your ability. As we progress through the following months, you will update your progress. Make sure to keep your journal in a safe place or saved on your hard drive. Use pictures as documentation as well. Take a picture of yourself standing from the front and from the side, and then an aerial shot from above you when you are measuring your injury.

No Judgement

This is a tool for measure and progress, not a tool to discourage or disqualify your feelings. There is not "right" or "wrong," just a measurement.

Yes, you can do this. If your injury feels like a cavern today, you can do this. If your injury is 20 years old, you can do this. If a woman with a 24 centimeter tear can self repair through this system, you can. If a grandmother in her 60's can self repair through this, you can. There is no limit to what you can do unless you place limits on your own progress. Just remember that!

Hernia

It is possible that through the process of getting this injury, or in the delicate days before you knew you had an injury, that the umbilical cord got trapped in the space between the halves of the rectus abdominis.

Sometimes, a piece of intestine can get stuck, as well. Sometimes, you can feel a hard protrusion in the space. If you can feel something in the space, get your hernia diagnosed by a physician or specialist. Ask for a definitive answer, not a "maybe." Some professionals call "Diastasis Recti" a "hernia" and do not differentiate between the two. You need to know whether there is just a space between halves of the muscle, or if there is a protrusion or hinderance to your healing. An intestinal hernia, if trapped, can be an emergency. If there is a protrusion through your muscle that you can feel or is causing pain, seek immediate medical help and insist on a definitive answer. "Is this a Diastasis, a hernia, or both? What are your conclusive measurements of the injury/hernia?"

In my experience, you cannot exercise out a hernia, but you CAN close the gap around the hernia. Your physician will talk to you about his recommendation based on his experience with hernia like yours. Your doctor may or may not recommend surgery. If he recommends surgery, consider doing your very best with the methods outlined in this book before the surgery so that the surgery itself is minimal.

Chapter 5:

The ABC's

This lesson changes everything.

This is instant relief, and the most important step you will take in healing your Diastasis Recti or other core and back problems. You remember the ABC's of the alphabet, right? Learning those ABC's led to reading words, sentences, paragraphs, and books. If you had never learned your ABC's, how advanced would your reading skills be?

These ABC's are the alphabet for core healing, and the foundation for everything we do here.

The ABC's for core healing: A is for Alignment, B is for Breathing, and C is for Core Engagement.

A = Alignment

Your mom was right in the sixth grade when she told you to stand up straight and stop slouching. Not only does it make you look and act more confident, but sitting and standing with good posture reduces pain, relieves symptoms, and helps you heal, all at once.

I say "all at once," and what I mean is "have patience and give yourself grace." This is because, depending on how much time you have been out of alignment, you may find re-aligning yourself is difficult and maybe even a little uncomfortable.

The discomfort you may feel is from using muscles that may have been sitting dormant for a while, or even from resetting your skeleton, which tends to morph to how you hold it. This is the part where your chiropractor thanks me for bringing this to your attention. Your mom will thank me, too.

Do This:

Take a picture of your full frame from head to foot. Take another one from the side. It helps to have a partner help you with this.

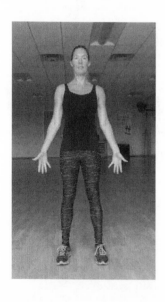 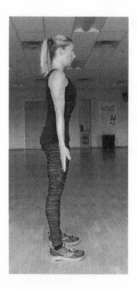

Look at your pictures and line up your parts.

From the side, you should have in a straight line:

1. Crown of the head
2. Top of the ear
3. Shoulder
4. Base of the ribs
5. Top of the pelvis
6. Hip joint
7. Knee
8. Ankle

From the front, notice the length of your neck, and whether your shoulders are even. If your neck looks short, you might be protruding your head forward or holding your shoulders high.

Now, we're going to start resetting your posture and alignment. It may be uncomfortable at first, and it will actually take practice to maintain.

Your crown sits on the top back part of your head, over your ears, like you're looking straight forward, not down or up. Press up through the crown of your head. For most people, that means pulling the chin in and lengthening the back of the neck, which is the top of your spine.

To practice proper shoulder placement, squeeze them first too high, up by your ears. Then, push them all the way back. Then push them down and hold them in place. For now, open your palms to the front. It helps set the shoulder.

Doing all of that may have set your ribcage forward, so use the top of your abdominal wall to pull your ribs in so that the ribs lay flat across the front and over your pelvis, not in front of your pelvis.

Push down through the base of your spine. Don't tuck your tailbone like a scorned puppy. Just press the base down slightly. You will feel an engagement happen in the front of the body, around the navel and pelvis. The two points to notice here are the top of the pelvis and the actual hip joint. They should be in direct line.

Finally, the legs are directly under the hip bones.

Take a new picture. How did you do?

Are you afraid to move? Don't be. You will be able to walk and move once you get the hang of those important points. When you sit down, sit as if you're standing. When you're moving around, be conscious of the length of your spine. Use your legs and hips to bend and move, rather than slumping down with your spine. Set up your work station so that you can sit up straight. If you are breastfeeding, set up a breastfeeding station that cushions you and supports your arms so that you can sit up straight, or lie down supported.

Like I said, this may be exhausting at first. It takes practice. Give yourself grace. Take breaks. The best way to take breaks is to sit in a chair with a back, lie on your back, or lean against a wall. The best way to practice is to have an hourly reminder on your phone, or to adjust every time you pass a window or mirror.

Did you notice a difference from the first to the second picture? Do you look instantly taller and slimmer? Yes, posture does that, too. It gives the appearance of a more long and lean physique, and can help you enter a room with confidence! If you have been struggling with pain and discomfort anywhere in your body, start to take notes on your pain level. You may find that this alone has solved many of your problems.

Example: one-minute posture adjustment

This is Amy Katherine, showing how much she could change her alignment in one minute. You can see how

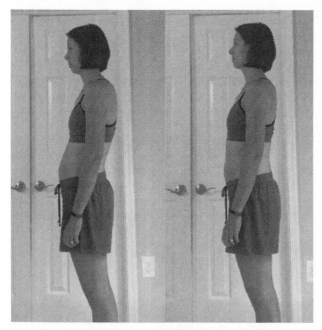

Much that changes the entire body!

B = Breathing

The next part to tackle is how to breathe properly. Most of us were taught to belly breathe for relaxation, or we have defaulted to a shallow, high chest breath.

Remember my story about coming out of surgery and feeling like I was suffocating? When the nurse was telling me to breathe, all I knew how to do was belly breathe, and I couldn't, so I could not get enough oxygen. This practice will be a practice, too. Give yourself grace to learn what could be a brand new breathing technique. This is not MY design. This was designed by Joseph Pilates, who cured his own Asthma with this technique and helped many soldiers heal from injury and ailment in World War I. Yes, THAT Pilates.

Your lungs live under your ribcage. At the base of your lungs is an involuntary muscle called the diaphragm.

Starting today, you will breathe into your actual lungs, where they live. To practice, put your hands on your ribs. They go all the way around your trunk, covering your lungs. As you breathe in, you will expand your lungs all the way around, NOT your belly. As you exhale, you simply expel the air evenly, still not pushing out through the abdominal walls.

Imagine as you breathe in that you can pull your navel up and under your rib cage while you expand your lungs all the way around. As you exhale, keep the navel lifted. This is not a shoulder exercise, so keep the shoulders down and in the shoulder girdle, as we described in the alignment section. Do not round your spine. Keep pressing up through the top of your head and down through the base of your spine, keeping your alignment the same. Just expand your lungs and release the air. Also, do not open your rib cage to the front. Keep your ribs all in line, expanding all the way around.

Having trouble? Don't hyperventilate. Don't shock your system. Breathe at a pace that feels right to you and give yourself the grace to figure this out. If you find that this is a very difficult new practice for you, take five minutes three times a day to focus just on that piece. You can do it!

C = Core Engagement

Along with these two principles comes core engagement. That feeling of the navel pulling up and in that happened when you aligned yourself is core engagement. That feeling when you were breathing and pulling the navel up and in is also core engagement. What we need to practice now is intentional, consistent core engagement.

Core engagement is not squeezing the tummy muscles, and it's not a vacuum of the abdominal walls. It feels like a flattening and holding of the abdominal muscles up and in. This is your CORE of support. This is the support system for your back and your organs, so it's very important.

Draw the navel up and in. The feeling around your pelvis is like zipping up a pair of pants that is one size too small. Hold your muscles in gently, like your abdominals are a hammock, holding your organs up and in. Keep the ribs tucked so that they are in line with your pelvis. Keep the engagement in the inhale and the exhale, never pushing the abdominal wall outward.

As you practice the alignment, breathing, and core engagement working together, you may feel like it is not cooperating at first. That is ok. It is a practice. Again, make intentional time, especially in the morning as you set your day, to practice these three principles. Be consistent and it will pay off. The muscle discomfort will ease and you will notice that your back may even look more toned! Keep practicing, but don't stop moving forward in the book. The rest of the book will help you stay consistent in this practice.

If you get stuck, go back to the beginning of this ABC practice. Take your time, and work toward getting just a few minutes of focus at a time. It will get easier!

Follow along with me as we practice the ABC's in this Video Series, a 4 part **BONUS** for joining me in this book. Get started Here: https://tinyurl.com/CarrieFitVideoSeries

Chapter 6

Do's and Don'ts (For Now)

You just found out that you have some element of an injury, and you are working on the ABC basics of healing. While that healing is happening on the inside of you, we have to treat this like an injury. If you had injured your rotator cuff, you would not be pitching the next softball game. If you had injured your meniscus, you would not be playing tackle football right now.

The same idea applies to your abdominal injury. We would not want to put additional stress on that part of your body while it is healing.

Basics for Life Right Now:

You have learned how to align yourself while sitting, standing, or lying. Adhere to this general alignment rule. If you are carrying people or things, continue to keep your spine aligned and your core engaged. For instance, when you pick something up, you will squat, using your legs, and lift that person or thing with leg and arm strength. You will not stoop over, hunching your back and allowing that alignment to fall. Keep in mind any time you lift something that if it becomes too heavy for you, your abdominals will try to "help" you by pushing outward. This only inhibits your recovery, and you should absolutely avoid lifting to that level of strain. You may need to enlist some help for a little while for heavy objects.

Do not round your back and droop your shoulders in order to bend down. Instead, bend from your knees and hips, supporting with your hands if you need to, to keep your spine in a long line and your core engaged.

Common Alignment Errors:

1. Jutting the hip to the side when holding something.
2. Jutting the abdominals forward, using them has a shelf
3. Jutting the pelvis forward while carrying something
4. Lifting with the back, rather than the legs.
5. Rounding the back to lift or move things.
6. Slouching while sitting (get a back on your chair or use a pillow for support)

Try to lift and move things from your shoulder level down. If you do have to reach on a high shelf for something, use a step stool, brace your core, and use your arm strength to get it down. Do not yank your body weight upward or let someone pull your arm up to pick you up. That is a lot of pressure on the sensitive area around the upper rectus abdominis and can cause your injury to open more.

Avoid twisting from the center of your body. Depending on your injury, you can move laterally somewhat, but large twisting motions from the center of the body, especially when moving an object with weight or density, is stressful on the abdominals. If you have a significant injury, you can feel the halves of the rectus abdominis shifting against each other in lateral and twist movements. This is not helpful in healing. Instead, use your legs and hips to twist from side to side, keeping the integrity of spinal alignment.

Example A: Twisting from the body's center. Not advised.

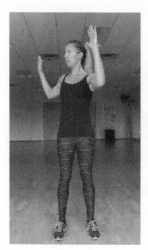 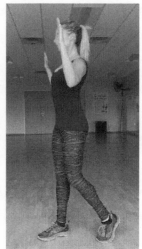

A.   B.

Example B: Twisting from the hips and legs. This is a
better choice for now.

When moving from standing to sitting or sitting to
standing, make sure to keep your core engaged and use
the strength of your legs and arms. It helps to align
yourself before standing up to avoid crunching the
abdominals to stand.

When moving from sitting to lying or lying to sitting, turn on to your side and use your arms to push yourself up or down. Do not lie on your back and sit straight up or flop onto your back from a seated position.

Special Situations

Breastfeeding

Breastfeeding should be a comfortable situation for you and baby. Quite often, you may find yourself in less-than-best situations when feeding a child. However, whenever possible, use a designated station that has plenty of pillows. You don't want to hunch over baby to breastfeed or use your abdominals as a baby seat. Adjust your seating and pillows so that you can sit up or lie on your side and nestle the baby comfortably.

Baby Carrying

Many people use front and back baby carriers as a great way to stay close to baby and keep hands free. Make sure to use a baby carrier that has a strap across the lower back for support. If you find that you are slumping to carry the baby or it becomes a burden on your back or tummy, consider a support band. My recommendation is listed in Chapter 8.

Mom Stuff

As a parent, you will be carrying a lot of stuff: bags, baby carriers, fold up strollers, etc. The best case scenario is to have a plan. You should not be carrying more than your limbs can handle at any given time. If you find yourself in a pinch, just do the best you can, keep yourself aligned and engaged, and take breaks.

Baby carriers are very hard to carry properly. Stay upright and hold it to one side, or use both hands and hold it to the front.

When getting the car seat in and out of the car, prop your foot inside of the car so that your leg can be supporting the weight. When getting children and babies in and out of the car, use the same process or sit in the back seat for a moment while assisting a child.

Fitness

Just like with any injury, we need to adjust your fitness life for now. We do not want you to stop exercising altogether, but we need to adjust how we do things. You will learn in subsequent chapters some specific exercises that encourage healing. This section is for safety. You want to be in better shape, not wreck your progress during your workout.

First of all, do not lift more weight than you can control following your rules of alignment, breathing, and core engagement. Some people will want to use waist trainers or tight girdles to keep the abdominal walls together. I have to warn you that those products cause other internal issues, including pelvic floor problems. The only garment should be a support garment. The one I recommend is in Chapter 8. Do not cinch your waist, and do not fall prey to the "push out" rule commonly passed around gyms. You should never push your abdominals out, especially when lifting weights.

Just like in our life lessons, be aware of how you are performing leg exercises. Keep proper alignment and form. Breathe and engage the way we have discussed. Keep the abdominals away from the thighs, like they are repelling magnets.

In any kind of plank exercise, including dolphin plank, push ups, side planks, burpees, and bird dogs, at least one knee must be down.

Modified example:

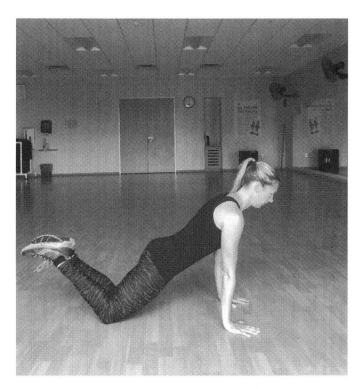

Just like in life, when moving from seated to lying or lying to seated, roll on to your side first, using your arms to adjust your positioning. When lying on your back, or "supine," do not lift your head. Only lift one foot at a time.

Just like in life, twist from your hips, not your abdomen. This includes dancing. Do not do lateral oblique exercises, like side crunches.

Do not attempt to push or pull weight above your shoulder line. In other words, when lying on your back, do not pull a weight over your head. When sitting or standing, do not perform pull downs or pull ups. Do not hang from an overhead bar.

When sitting or standing, lift only one foot or leg at a time. Consider this when running or adding high impact activities. It takes a lot of core engagement to leave the ground. Doing it properly takes a lot of practice and some level of healing. Consider taking out impact for right now, until you have a secure hold on how running or jumping will impact your core and organs. Many people experience abdominal swelling from running or jumping, because the abdominal wall is just not able to support the internal organs yet. We will talk about how to add it back in later. For now, try low impact exercise.

Swimming is also difficult to support. Let's consider swimming after we have mastered the art of alignment, breathing, and core engagement.

I have given you a lot of rules and a lot to think about. Here is the bottom line: if it feels like it's pressure on the core, stop. Revisit your alignment, breathing, and core engagement. Adjust and modify.

Summary/ Basic modification list:

- Put One knee down in any kind of plank
- When on your back, keep your head and shoulders down
- Lift one leg at a time
- No shoulder exercises above the shoulder line
- Roll onto your side when moving from seated-lying or lying-seated

You may have to explain yourself for a while to your instructor or trainer. Offer this book as a guide if they want to help you. Most trainers do not know exactly what your modifications will look like, so help teach him or her what you need. In a fitness class, you may be doing things the other people are not doing. Remember that you are in this to heal, not just to fit in with the rest of the class. Instructors and other members should respect that you have a different plan for right now. If nothing else, the fact that you are empowered with this knowledge can help others. Many people in your class are probably struggling with the same problem. Be your own best advocate and help others with their voices, as well.

For example:

- Everyone else is jumping. I am stepping.
- Everyone else is twisting from their waist. I am turning my feet to twist from my legs.
- Everyone else is doing burpees. I am doing lunges.

- Everyone else is doing pull-ups. I am doing supported rows.
- Everyone else is doing push-ups. I have my knees down.
- Everyone else is doing sit ups. I am doing bridges.
- Everyone else is doing double leg lifts. I am doing single leg lifts.

Chances are, you will inspire someone else to modify for their own health, too. Fitness is not about fitting in. It is about getting better and stronger in your own skin.

Chapter 7:

Mind-Body Connection

Here is the part of the book where many of you are going to want to shut the book or just call me crazy. Something in you might hesitate or get frustrated. Stay with me. This is the part that we have to discuss mind-body connection in core healing.

Most of my life, even as kinesthetically aware as I am, I was not mentally connected to how my muscles worked, especially my core muscles. This was amplified when I had my first baby. Looking back now, I was practically numb below the neck. I didn't recognize my own body.

Fast forward to a surgery that ripped apart muscle and nerves, and I was literally numb, as well as traumatized. It took me long, frustrating hours of focus and meditation to finally feel what core engagement and muscle contraction actually feel like.

As I talk with women every day, I find that my story is not the exception but the rule. Many women went through some kind of trauma around childbirth or in their postpartum life, including lack of recognition of their bodies in the mirror. Many women have been cut by a knife during delivery. Many struggled with their pregnant bodies. Many more are practically in a state of shock after birth, because of their own image of what post-birth "should" look like in their mind's eye. The difference in expectation and reality can be monumental.

Therapist Alexis Edwards in Austin, Texas, says that an old trauma can resurface at or after childbirth, due to raw emotions and extreme life changes. Understandably, this can greatly impact a woman's connection to her body.

Let's take a moment for you to find your mind-body connection. First of all, how easy or difficult was the ABC method? Did the breathing not connect with you right away? When I asked you to feel that core pull up and in, did you FEEL it? Did you get frustrated? Did you think you were alone in feeling this way?

You're Not Alone. This is a practical practice in re-engaging your mind and your body. It might feel weird or very woo-woo at first, especially if meditation is not part of your practice. We are not looking for an altered state. We are looking to be fully present in the body that we are in. So, bear with me.

You may want to read this section first and then close your eyes to practice feeling things internally. Some people find this to be helpful, and some want to just look at the words or a simple image while they focus. There is no "wrong" in finding your connection within. Just practice with me.

Let's start with the easiest places to feel energy and life. I know, I know, this sounds like a new age method of transcendence, but I assure you, it's for you to be successful in your mission of healing.

Start by rubbing your hands together. Can you feel one hand on the other? Can you feel just your right hand? Can you feel just your left hand? Now, lay your hands on your lap and focus on just feeling the life in your hands. There is energy in there. Can you feel it, just sitting still? Science tells us that we are vibrating all the time. This is a practice to find that vibration.

Now practice feeling the energy and life in your feet. As you focus on your feet, can you feel the life going through them? Imagine blood flowing through your arms and legs, and find the life and energy in them as well.

Now is the tough part. We are going to find that life energy in our torso. Take a moment to put your hand on your chest. Notice your heart pumping and your chest moving as you breathe. Feel your lungs expand all the way into your armpits and into your shoulders and into your back.

In your abdominal area, try some mini-muscle contractions. Remember that we always want the muscles to flex inward, so take a moment and draw your navel up and in. Release that without pushing the muscle back out. Now think lower. Think about flattening your lowest abdominal muscles, around the pelvis. Pull that muscle up and in. Release it without pushing it out. Now feel your breath and your muscles working together to stabilize your body. Feel your muscles wrap you all the way around your midsection. Take a moment to appreciate that they hold you together and protect your vital organs.

Put one hand on your chest and the other on your stomach area. Feel the muscles of the abdomen pull up and in while the ribs expand as you take a breath in. Feel the muscles of the abdomen stay contracted while you expel air from your lungs.

In yoga, we consider the internal, intuitive observer to be the "third eye." You may or may not want to consider your mind's eye to be your third eye, but if it helps, use it. If you just want to use your internal knowing, that is fine, too. Take your internal knowing or third eye to the center of your body. Watch and feel everything working together. Feel what you feel. Some things may surface, or you may get frustrated with areas that seem blocked or numb. Just know that this is part of the process, and have patience as your mind finds your body again.

If some emotions are coming up for you, experience them and breathe through it. There is no wrong way to feel as you go through this process. If it is bringing up specific trauma, however, I encourage you to seek counsel immediately.

Remember through this and all of the processes we are using here that you are in charge of your body. You deserve the time to heal. You deserve to feel well. You deserve to feel loved from within. You deserve to feel strong. You deserve to take care of you. Only when you care for yourself can you really show up as your best self for everyone else. Take the time you need to heal, don't rush yourself, and trust your process.

Remember that you grew a human life inside of you, which makes you a superhero. Remember that the body was created to create, and that it was also created to heal. Our body tissue rehabilitates and reconstructs itself all day every day. This is the same process, we are just encouraging it to do so. We are mindful moving forward so that the body has a positive healing experience.

Before you leave this chapter, take 5 minutes and consider all of the things about you that make you strong enough to do this. What have you survived? What have you mastered? What have you pushed through? Show gratitude for the birthing experience that taught you and molded this part of your life. Show gratitude to your personal experiences that have led you right here right now.

What does this have to do with healing? Everything. Numbness is a block, and feeling is the key to self-healing. If you're struggling with a personal emotional trauma, seek counsel. If this has stirred something in you, work through that or have a specialist help you work through it. But be brave enough and bold enough to stand up for yourself. Understand that you are here on purpose for purpose. Persevere for the sake of your life and the lives around you. Your closest circle depends on it. Don't think that caring just for them and not yourself does anyone any good. Your care for YOU is the catalyst for care for everyone around you.

Let's turn mindfulness into a conscious practice. This works best in a quiet space, and for many mothers, that is really hard to find. But even in the 1 minute you have when your child is sleeping, find your time to close your eyes and breathe, or open your eyes to the space that surrounds you and just focus on being.

You don't need to be something or someone in particular. Just Be Here Now. Focus on life, breath, and feeling, even just for a few seconds, and notice if things start to open for you.

Chapter 8

Recommendations

This section is a handy guide for recommendations while you are working through this injury. First of all, recognize that you have an injury, and treat it like an injury. The previous chapters have given you some guidelines around work, home, and fitness. Please adhere to the guidelines to the best of your ability because your injury depends on it.

If you have a star athlete team with a torn muscle, are you playing her in the championships ? Later, yes. Today, no. Today, we take care of her first. The same thing applies here. We want you to be the best at what you do, so for right now, that means treating your injury like an injury and treating yourself with some basic self care.

Move.

Don't stop moving just because you have an abdominal injury. If you stop moving altogether, you are creating another level of effect that is not serving you. Being inactive causes muscles to atrophy, decreases cardiovascular function, and can increase risk of respiratory problems, heart issues, and general weakness that lead to more injury.

Instead of being fearful of movement, take the guidelines in the previous chapters and get out and move. Even a walk in the park is better than an afternoon on the couch. You CAN push your jogger stroller. Just do it with really good alignment, posture, and breathing. Go without the impact of jogging or running right now. It is still a workout, and it still will get your body moving and pumping blood, which is what you need.

Resistance exercises are as simple as squatting, bending from the hips, circling the arms, or any number of basic movements. In Chapter 9, you will get a series of strengthening exercises and even full body movements to use to stay fit while you are protecting and healing your injury.

Eat.

Many people with a protruding abdomen go back to the old story " I'm fat," and some people have even been TOLD by professionals that the problem is fat, not seeing the underlying issue. Do yourself a favor and stop seeing the problem as a fat problem. Start seeing yourself with an injury that you are working to heal.

If your child was sick or hurt, would you stop feeding her? No! You know that a sick or injured child needs nutrients in order to heal and get better. Even when she doesn't feel well, you're going to make her chicken soup and encourage her to try a piece of fruit, right?

Why would you treat yourself any differently? Starving yourself or depriving yourself of nutrition will not solve your problem. It will only set you back and hinder your progress.

Protein

Let's talk about the nutrition that would be most appropriate to you right now with this injury. The following recommendations are based on a study by Springer Sports Medicine, Australia, on the effects of foods on sports injuries.
(https://www.ncbi.nlm.nih.gov/pmc/articles/PMC4672013/)

The Springer Sports Medicine research was based on protein and a specific amino acid called creatine in injury recovery. The injuries researched were sports-based, but are applicable, I believe, because Diastasis Recti is a muscle and soft tissue injury that actually CAN be sports-related. The general protein recommendation from the study is roughly 2 grams of protein per day per kilogram of your personal body weight.

Let's do the math, especially for the Americans, who measure weight in pounds. One kilogram equals 2.2 pounds (you can do a simple google search for a pounds to kilos calculator if you prefer). Therefore, a 150 pound woman would be 68 kilograms in weight, multiplied by 2 equals 136 grams of protein per day. If she eats 3 times a day, she needs approximately 45 grams of protein per meal OR can use a protein supplement at some time during the day. I recommend Shakeology, which has 15 grams of protein, or Beachbody Recover (used post-exercise), which has 20 grams of protein. This helps with your total for the day.

Here are some protein sources to consider. Remember that the more whole and natural the food, the higher quality nutrition. Try to avoid processed foods and fast food as quick protein. Many quick fixes are also loaded with added sugar, salt, and fat.

Eggs (6g ea)

Almonds (6g/ounce)

Chicken Breast (around 50 g for one breast)

Plain Oats (15g/1/2 cup)

Cottage Cheese (15 g / cup)

Plain Greek Yogurt (17g / ½ cup)

Broccoli (3g/cup)

Beef Sirloin (22g / 3 ounce)

Tuna (39g/ cup)

Quinoa (8g / cup)

Lentils (18g/cup)

Pumpkin Seed (5g/ounce)

Brussel Sprouts (2g/1/2 cup)

Explore with all kinds of nuts and vegetables to find hidden gems of protein.

Creatine is a special amino acid that the body makes naturally. The research from the Springer Sports Medicine Group suggests that adding additional creatine to your diet may help your muscle and tissue repair from injury. If you do decide to supplement with Creatine, consider the Beachbody Creatine Supplement, as it is a pure, tasteless form of the amino acid. With any choice, make sure it is a clean, plain supplement. It should be tasteless. Like any other addition or supplement, take just the recommended daily allowance. Taking too much of any amino acid does not multiply its effects and can lead to an imbalance of amino acids.

Fats

Omega 3 fatty acids are also linked to tissue repair. I recommend having some source of omega 3 in your daily diet. Examples would be in fish and nuts. We do have to be careful not to over-consume fish, as recent concerns are tied to fish and mercury, a metal you do not want lingering in your body and brain. The best sources of fish that historically have low mercury counts are sardines, wild salmon, haddock, hake, and tilapia. Nuts and seeds high in omega 3 fatty acids are walnuts, chia seeds, and flax seeds. Walnuts are healthiest raw and unsalted, and chia and flax seeds are better digested when they have been ground first (a coffee grinder will do the trick). If you find that you are not getting daily Omega-3 in your diet, consider supplementing with a clean, natural fish oil or krill oil. Take a supplement or add a serving of Omega-3 to your daily routine.

Antioxidants

Antioxidants are so popular right now, right? Every commercial, every journal, and every nutrition guide tells you to eat your antioxidants! Why? Well, these genius foods fight free radicals and strengthen your tissue. Free radicals are these crazy radical molecules that like to break apart other molecules to make themselves feel more whole (selfish jerks). The Antioxidant in your body will combat that crazy radical, saving your skin and tissue from literal destruction. He needs a cape.

So, yes, you need to have antioxidant foods in your life every single day. The densest forms of antioxidants are in dark colored berries, dark chocolate, and dark green vegetables. The color is key! The dense, deep, dark colors tells you there is serious activity going on in that food, from phytonutrition, the nutrition from the source itself, the sun. However, beware the false antioxidant. Never consume a genetically modified fruit or vegetable, because he is an imposter and will do very little, nutritionally. GMO fruits and vegetables at the market have a PLU in the United States that starts with a number 8, so check that little sticker on your produce. They are NOT required to be labeled in the United States other than with this first number, so check. Leave him be and warn your sister not to pick him up, either.

For best results, go organic. An organic fruit or vegetable has not been soaked in poison, as have most of our fruits and vegetables in the United States. Yes, we are being poisoned by our food every day, and it's totally legal. Organic produce in the market will have a 9 in the front of the PLU.

Dark chocolate, you say? Yes, I am telling you to eat 1 square of dark chocolate per day. The darker the better. Too much chocolate can start adding calories quickly, which is why I stick to one square a day. That one square a day may keep the doctor away! Put THAT on a poster somewhere.

For me personally, I drink a Shakeology every day. That all-food supplement drink has 70 super foods in it, including all the phytonutrients and antioxidants I need, and nothing I don't. So if you're like me and you don't shop at the market for your antioxidant foods on the daily, keep some Shakeology around the house. It's also incredibly tasty.

Now for the bad news. What HINDERS the reconstruction and repair of your tissue? Alcohol. I just saw you wince. For now, take my advice and pare back the wine and beer while you're healing. Processed foods and sugars will also weaken your body's natural ability to heal.

Skin

Your skin might feel loose right now. Some of that is from sudden changes in the skin, and some is from the muscles and tissue under the skin, making the skin appear stretched or wrinkled. Skin tightening and firming treatments haven't been proven on a postpartum belly, and many of the products and services marketed to women don't have any evidence of helping in this kind of skin. Ask your dermatologist or aesthetician what she recommends, and be patient in the process.

The healthiest skin comes from the inside out. Keep your body well-hydrated, starting with at least 60 ounces of water per day (not all at once). Healthy skin is also dependent upon the same nutrition we have already mentioned: a balance of protein, whole foods, and phytonutrients.

Other thoughts and recommendations:

Splinting

Many people ask about girdles, waist trainers, and splints when it comes to this injury. For the most part, I don't necessarily want you to use a device rather than your own muscle control. Training your muscles to hold yourself up and together is the backbone of this training. However, there may be instances where it becomes difficult to do so, and you may just feel like you need support. One time I definitely think you should use extra support, at least in the temporary time period, is baby-wearing. Wearing and carrying a baby puts a lot of long term pressure on the abdominal muscles, and after a while, it can be impossible to maintain good form. Sometimes, people feel like they need more support during exercise temporarily, and that is fine, too.

There is only one splint that I recommend currently (as of mid-2018), and it is by ReCore Fitness, called the Post Natal Fit Splint. You can find it here : https://www.recorefitness.com/store/p4/Post-Natal_FITsplint%E2%84%A2_.html
This splint is neoprene, covers the injury, and is very adjustable. When placing it, it should not feel like it is squeezing you. It should feel like it is supporting your existing efforts to stand straight and hold yourself upright.

Other products that advertise waist cinching I do not advise using. Anything that is squeezing you together is also squeezing your internal organs, which can cause pelvic floor issues in the short or long term. I have also had clients whose muscles were torn by waist trainers. If it feels like it's squeezing the life out of you, it probably is.

Doctor

When you discover that you have a level of Diastasis, it is not usually an emergency to see a physician. Usually, you can just start this program and start to feel better instantly, which takes away the immediate need for physical evaluation. However, if you are in pain, even after starting this program, if you're concerned that your injury is beyond Diastasis Recti, or you have something hard protruding out of your abdomen, see a physician. If you are humming along with this program, just let him know on your next physical examination that you think you have significant Diastasis Recti, and ask he can tell if you also have umbilical hernia. This is important to know because you can work your muscles back together, but you cannot completely exercise out a hernia. Depending on what he sees, he may recommend surgery. My recommendation in this circumstance and the recommendation of board certified plastic surgeon and friend Dr. Alina Sholar is to do this method, repair your own diastasis, and then only have the hernia itself repaired. A hernia repair is done by a general or plastic surgeon, is generally outpatient, and generally has a relatively easy recovery (remember that NO surgery is EASY). A Diastasis Surgery is intense plastic surgery, like what I wrote about in chapter 2, and it can take years or a lifetime to recover.

If you do decide to have the full Diastasis Recti Surgery (called an abdominoplasty), this same method will help you recover post surgery. So please come back to this book as you recover so that you can help yourself recover, but know that the recovery is a process.

Exercise

You have been given the fitness rules for a reason. You can self-modify your workouts to be safe for your body. You can go to your fitness center or workout at home. But please be an advocate for your own body. Do not let your trainer or coach tell you to do an exercise that you know is counter-intuitive to your healing. It is your job to do what is right for yourself You may find yourself educating and helping your fitness professionals. There are not very many professionals in the fitness space who really understand the depth of this injury, and many do not understand what they can do to help people modify. You can be the catalyst for helping others!

Chapter 9:

The Strength Series

The most important parts of your healing are the ABC's, discussed in Chapter 5, and how you lead your life, discussed in Chapters 6-8, but here, we want to strengthen the core stability muscles to help move your progress forward.

The best way to move forward with these exercises is to focus on each section, one at a time, one section per day, rotating through all of the sections for 6 weeks. You will do about 8-10 repetitions per exercise, depending on your engagement. As soon as you feel like you're losing engagement or strength, or if something hurts, cramps, or feels simple "wrong," give yourself a pass and come back to it in a couple of days.

The First word to remember in your healing? Consistency. Be slow and consistent to get the most reward.

The Second word to remember is Grace. You won't be perfect, and each day may feel different than the day before. Your body will tell you if it is too exhausted to go on or if it wants to try a little harder. Listen to it. Always go to the boundary of comfort, but never past the boundary and into pain. It should be focused and strong, not reckless or painful.

Before beginning your daily practice, go back to your ABC's and review. Align, Breathe, and Engage. I also recommend either going through the mind-body connection of Chapter 7 or having some kind of mindful moment before beginning each day. Even a very thoughtful breath can get you in the right mode for success.

Every Section in this chapter has an accompanying video, showing me performing a couple of reps of each exercise. Watch these to better understand your form and approximate speed, though your speed depends on your control (slow and steady) and your breath (fully inflate your lungs). Here is a link to get those videos: http://www.carriefit.com/fmppb-chapter-9-supplemental-videos/

Section 1: Supine

Lie on your back on the floor safely. It will be most comfortable on a firm but not hard surface. A mat over the floor will usually suffice. Remember not to roll down and up, but to use your hands and knees to get down to the floor and roll on to your side and then on to your back.

Exercise 1: Floor Positioning

Once you get to the floor on your back, lie with the back
of your head down, shoulder blades flat on the floor, hip
bones down, knees bent and feet flat on the ground.
Have a little space between your knees.

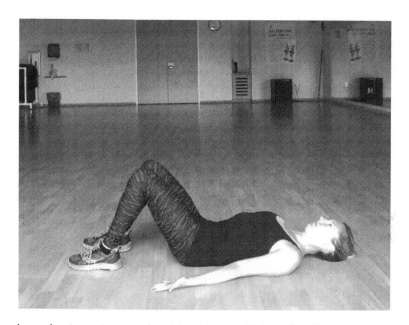

In order to get your shoulder blades flat on the floor, you
may need to have your palms up, or even bend your
elbows and let your hands come up. Don't skip this part.
Shoulders need to be far away from your ears and flat.

Make the back of your neck long. That is the top of your spine. Press through the top of your head, like we did when we were standing. Tuck your tailbone just enough so that the entire spine can touch the floor. Don't press it in to the floor, just a light touch is fine.

Start practicing breathing into your lungs. On the floor like this, it's easier to feel the air expand the lungs into your back. Make sure you're not raising your shoulders to breathe. Keep all of your ribs in line. Draw the navel up and in and you breathe, and keep it there to exhale. Be strong in both the inhale and exhale, but don't turn it into a vacuum exercise.

Pretend like you just zipped up a pair of pants one size too tight. That will help draw the area around the pelvis in, and draw the inner thighs upward in a light hold.

Did I give you enough to think about yet? Don't be afraid. It gets easier with practice. Give yourself time to ease into this important beginning station. Take a few breaths before moving on. Practice having a hand on your chest and the other on the abdomen, and remember that the navel should continually pull up and in while the ribs expand and contract.

Exercise 2: Pelvic Tilt

From the supine position, tuck your tailbone 2 extra inches until it comes off the floor. It should be like peeling your tailbone up. As you do this, exhale and focus on the flatness of the lowest abdominal muscles, right around the pelvis. Take a breath at the top, peel the tailbone back down as you exhale.

The exhale is in the moving. The inhale is in the stillness. This movement is also very important for your practice. Be very mindful in what you are doing, really tucking up and pulling the navel up, not just using your hips. The front body and back body have to work together, all from the transverse abdominis, which surrounds your core.

Exercise 3: Bridge

Start with your pelvic tilt and begin to peel the next part of the spine up from the bottom. Keep peeling until you are straight from shoulders to knees. Make sure the pelvis is still tilted under. Take a breath. Exhale as you set the spine back down from top to bottom. Try your best to set each piece of your spine down as if it were painter's tape and you don't want an air bubble in it. Take more time where you have stiffness. At the top of this exercise, make sure you still have the ribs tucked in line with you, not arching your back. You are a straight line from shoulders to knees.

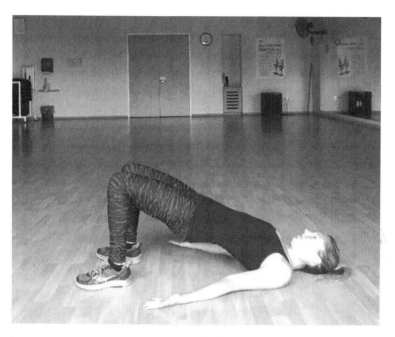

In your next set of bridge, hold your inner thighs and knees together. This isometric hold is important for stabilizing the area around the pelvic floor and transverse abdominis. A nice side effect is a stronger pelvic floor area.

Exercise 4: Single Leg Press

Come back down to the floor with knees still bent. Engage your core and bring your right knee up so that the knee is directly over the hip bone and the knee is in a 90 degree angle. Make sure you spine is still all the way on the floor.

Put your hands stacked on your thigh muscles, just above your knee. Without moving, push your hands on your thigh and your thigh on your hands. Push as hard as you can from both directions but DON'T MOVE. Exhale for a count of 3. Place the right foot down and repeat the exercise on the left.

Exercise 4: Single Leg March

Before beginning this exercise, take a break. Let your legs lay out long. Your spine can lift off of the mat. Let your hips and legs shake, roll, and move. Allow your spine to lift slightly, just enough to elongate the muscles you have been using.

Now come back to your supine position with knees bent. Bring your right knee over your right hip bone, with your leg in a 90 degree angle. Put your hands on your abdomen. Take a breath as you hinge from your hip bone to lower your foot toward the ground. This is about the hip joint, not the knee and ankle joint. The movement should be only from the hip. Stop at the boundary where it feels like your back is going to leave the mat, or where your abdomen is about to push outward. Do NOT let it push outward. Exhale as you return to the starting position. Complete your set on the right and then do the same set on the left. Make sure to count your repetitions. If you can not do the same number on both sides, take note of that. Sides of the body may act differently. We will be working toward balance.

Exercise 5: Single Leg Pendulum

Lay the legs out straight on the floor and the arms straight out to the sides, in line with the shoulders, palms facing up.

Bend the right knee and bring it over the hip bone in a 90 degree angle. The difference now is that the lower back might not be on the floor. What is important here is the core engagement and keeping the ribs down. Pelvis will stay glued down, not rocking side to side, and both shoulder blades stay flat down on the floor.

The left leg is planted down into the ground, with toes flexed upward. It is there to stabilize you. Bring your right knee across the midline of your body as you exhale. Do not lift either hip off of the floor. The hips and left leg remain flat, still, and on the floor. Inhale as you open the knee away from the midline of the body, stopping before you lift the hips or lose engagement. Continue by exhaling to bring the knee across again. Complete your set on the right, then set the right foot down, lay it out, and begin the process with the left leg.

Section 2: Prone Position

Today, you will lay down flat on the floor on your belly. Start by getting to your hands and knees, and then lower yourself down. Fold your hands one over the other and lay your forehead on your hands, right in the center. Make the back of your neck long. Press your shoulders deep down your back. Tuck your tailbone under you until you feel your core engage and navel drawing away from the floor. This is an important practice. At no time in this practice will we want the navel to push into the floor. This limits your range of motion, and that is just fine. Thighs are strong, like you're lifting your knees up.

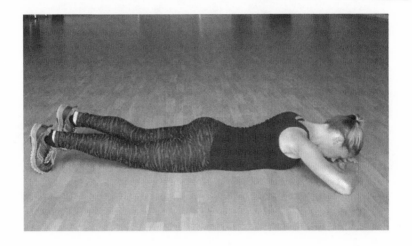

Practice breathing in this position. You will definitely feel the front of your ribs expand. Practice getting the air into your sides and back without losing the navel lift. Keep the front of the pelvis facing the mat.

Exercise 1: Elbow raise

Without losing this form, exhale as you lift your elbows, and inhale as they return to the floor. Do not shrug your shoulders. Keep the back of your neck (upper spine) nice and long. Press your shoulders down your back as you lift.

Exercise 2: Single leg raise

Let the elbows stay on the floor and keep your alignment. Nail the front of your pelvis down to the ground. Do not rock side to side.

As you exhale, lengthen and lift your right leg. Imagine it getting longer, even if it doesn't go very high.
Remember, we are keeping the bones of the front of the pelvis flat to the front and the spine nice and long. Inhale to return the right leg, and then exhale to lift the left. Continue a slow, mindful pattern.

Exercise 3: Single arm-Single leg cross body raises

Keeping your head in line with your spine, or by replacing your hands with a rolled-up cloth, bring your arms to a 90 degree angle by your sides, with elbows in line with the shoulders. Raise the right arm and left leg at the same time without rotating the body or lifting the hips. The shoulder is pressing down the back and the leg is lengthening away from the spine.

Alternate sides and watch out for rocking. Keep the head stabilized.

Section 3: Side-lying series

Lie on your left arm. Lengthen that arm so that your head can rest down on your bicep. Do NOT prop your head on your hand. We are looking for a long, straight spine. Tuck your shoulder under you, not up by your ear. Elongate the spine. Tuck your tailbone under you and bend your knees slightly. Try to make your spine as long as possible from neck to tailbone. Imagine that you are wearing a tight corset from ribs to hips. Flatten the pelvic floor area, like you zipped it up a little too tight. Feel the navel pull up and in. Pull the side body out of the floor. If your side body is pushing down into the floor, check your spinal alignment again. You should have shoulder over shoulder, ribs lined up, hip over hip, knee over knee, and foot over foot. This alignment may take practice the first time. Place your right hand on the floor in front of you for stability.

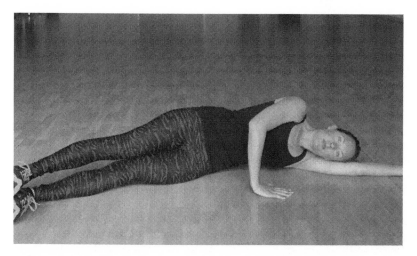

The whole purpose of this series is to stay aligned and avoid rotation. You do not want your hips or shoulders to rock back and forth or for your torso to move around.

Keep everything from head to hips firm and still. Got it? Easier said than done, I know.

Complete all of these side-lying exercises lying on your left side, and then move to lying on your right side and repeat.

Exercise 1: Side lying bent knee

Lift your right leg up so that your leg is even with your hip bone and parallel with the floor. Exhale to bend from the hip joint to bring the knee in front of you. Inhale to bring the leg back in line or even slightly behind you. Remember: your purpose is not rotating the hips or moving the torso.

Exercise 2: Opposing limbs

Straighten the right leg. Release your right arm from holding the ground.

As you exhale, bring your left leg in front of you while bringing your right arm behind you.

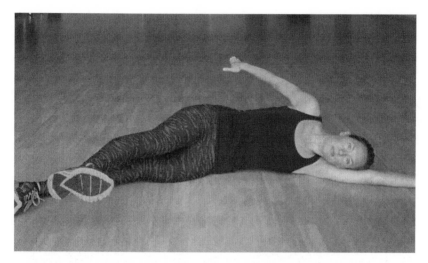

Inhale to bring your leg behind and your arm to the front. Again, the purpose is stability. Do not rock the torso or hips forward and back. Keep the hips and shoulders stacked.

Exercise 3: Knee to Elbow

Stack your legs. Bring your right arm over your head. Turn your toes slightly toward the ceiling, without losing your stacked hip alignment. Bend your right knee, sliding your toe toward your knee. Bring your knee up and toward your arm, while bringing your arm down and toward your knee. This form is easier if you keep your weight forward, as to avoid the backward shift.

Section 4: Quadruped

This section is from hands and knees. Start with your hands under your shoulders and your knees under your hips, slightly separated. Flex your feet. Spread your fingers out and hold your inner arms close to your sides. Lift out of the shoulder joint and tuck the tailbone until you can easily hold your lower back up and pull your navel up and in. The exercises will only help you if you maintain a flat back and keep your core muscles engaged. These are not intended to just be leg exercises. Keep your weight on your feet more than your hands.

If you have wrist or shoulder problems, you can do these same exercises with your elbows and forearms on the mat. Keep your forearms parallel to each other and your shoulders away from your ears.

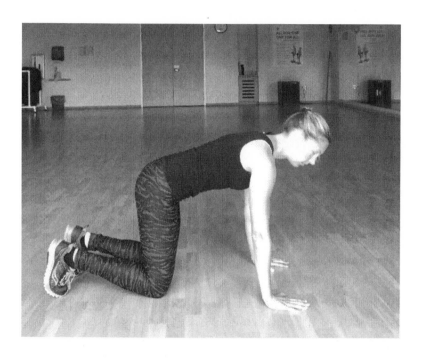

Exercise 1: Isometric feet pressing

Without moving or changing form, push most of your weight onto your feet. Hold as you exhale, release to inhale.

Exercise 2: Single leg stretch

Alternate sides with this exercise. Press your weight onto your right leg, sliding your toe back until your knee is straight. This is easier in socked feet or with a paper plate under your toes. Do not shift your body around, simply press back and straighten the leg as you exhale. Inhale to replace the knee to the ground.

Exercise 3: Fire hydrants

Keeping your weight evenly distributed in your hands and left leg, lift your right leg (keeping it bent) out to the side as you exhale. Do not twist the spine or open the hips to the side. Keep the shoulders in place. Inhale and lower the leg.

Exercise 4: Single arm raises

Exhale to raise one arm in front of you, to shoulder height. Do not change your shoulder or spine positioning. Alternate arms.

Exercise 5: Bird Dog

Bring the right arm out in front of you as you bring the left leg straight behind you and inhale. Use the leg that is on the ground for the majority of your weight and support. Keep your lower back elevated and hips squared off toward the ground, not rotated to the side. Exhale to lower your limbs. Alternate sides without rocking your body from side to side or swiveling hips.

Exercise 6: Half Plank

Start walking your knees back and continue tucking your tailbone under. The goal is a straight line from shoulder to knee, but you should stop when you start to feel yourself losing core engagement, or you feel your lower back or shoulders dropping. Hold for a breath, then take a break in child's pose for a moment.

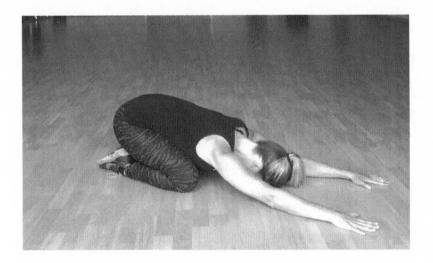

Section 5: Seated

Find yourself seated on the floor if possible. If you cannot sit on the floor, sit in a hard bottomed, sturdy chair where you can sit straight up and put your legs in a 90 degree angle from hips to knees to ankles.

If you are sitting on the floor, sit with the sits bones straight down on the floor, knees bent, and feet flat on the floor.

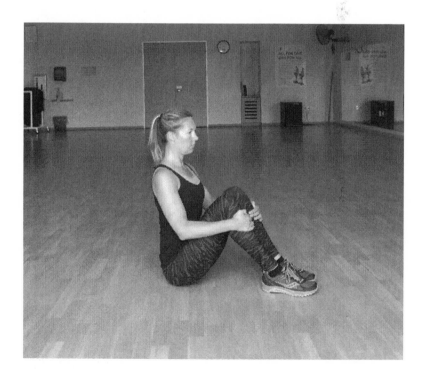

Exercise 1: Seated Isometrics

If you are on the floor, hold your shin bones with your hands without rounding your shoulders. Keep your spine all the way upright. If you are in a chair, put your hands on your thigh bones, above the knees.

Press legs and hands to each other as you exhale. Inhale to release. Focus on drawing the navel up and in, pulling the shoulders back and down, and pressing up through the back-top of your head.

Exercise 2: Single Leg Straightening

If you are seated on the floor, put your hands under the crease of your knee. If you are seated on a chair, put your hands on your thighs. Exhale as you straighten your right knee from the knee joint. Inhale as you bend it. Focus just on the right side for the first set and then on the left.

Exercise 3: Single Leg Lifts

If you are seated on the floor, straighten the legs out in front of you as much as you can while keeping your back upright and straight. This in itself is an exercise and can replace the movement for a while until your body is ready to move from this position.

If you are sitting, extend one leg straight and keep the other foot firmly planted on the floor. If it cannot lie flat on the floor, put a block or book under the foot to support you.

Focusing just on the right leg, lift and lower slowly. Exhale as you lift, inhale as you lower. If the leg does not move, just have the intention to move. This is a practice. Finish your set and then focus just on the left. Keep the sits bones down; just lift the leg itself.

Exercise 4: Spinal Flexion

From here, practice rounding the spine and then straightening back up. Exhale and draw the navel in to round or flex the spine and inhale to straighten.

Section 6: Standing

Stand by a sturdy wall. Place your feet under your hip bones, and follow the alignment instructions you learned in chapter 5.

Exercise 1: Wall Plank

Turn and face the wall. Put your hands directly out on the wall at your shoulder level. Start walking your feet back until you feel the weight shift onto your hands. Tuck your tailbone under more than you think you need to and draw the navel up. Return the feet to normal and repeat.

Exercise 2: Leg Swing

Turn to stand next to the wall. Put your hand on the wall next to you for support (as you get stronger, put your hand down and challenge your stability). Bend your knee until it is even with your hip bone to the front and exhale. Do not change your posture. Inhale as you lower the bent leg and bring your foot behind you. Again, do not change your posture or alignment. Finish your set and turn around to work the other side.

Exercise 3: Leg Pendulum

Still facing the side, put the leg furthest from the wall in front of you, toe touching the floor. Draw your navel up as you lift the straight leg. Exhale to bring the leg across the other leg and toward the wall. Inhale to bring the leg back across and out to the side. Do not shift your weight from side to side or change your spinal alignment. Complete one side, and then turn around to work the other side.

Exercise 4: Knee to elbow

Start by standing in your regular posture. Turn out the toe of the leg furthest from the wall. Bring the same arm over head. Exhale as you bring the knee and the elbow toward each other. Do not bend to make this happen. Keep your posture and alignment. Complete this side, and then turn around to complete the other side.

Exercise 5: Standing Hundreds

No wall or structure is necessary for this exercise. Stand with your hands by your thighs, palms facing behind you. Inhale to bring your arms straight in front of you, 6-8 inches, exhale as you press them behind you,

6-8 inches. The challenge is to make the movement big and quicken your pace, without shifting the weight of your body forward and back. Only move from the shoulder, not the spine.

Exit Protocol:

As you go through these exercises and use your modifications, you may be curious as to what to do next, or how to transition out of these exercises and modifications. There is no quick answer for this. Every injury is different. Time of healing is different. The way each body heals is different. As you start to see and feel improvement in your injury, doing your check once a month and journaling, as you find that your injury is not all the way through the muscle, that you can feel a layer under the muscle supporting you and healing, and the sides of the injury are touching or almost touching, then you will want to take the exit protocol quiz.

With the exit protocol, you will find which modifications you need to continue, and which ones you can start to ease out of. By easing out, we give ourselves permission to TRY an exercise, and to return to the modification as soon as we feel we are losing control or form.

By the time you take the Exit Protocol, you will be more in tune with what feels right or wrong in your own body, and can then take the precautions needed while exploring what you CAN do again.

I recommend reviewing your exit protocol every six weeks during your healing process.

Level 1: Full Plank

Go into the half plank exercise from the Quadruped Series. Push your weight back onto your feet. Start to lift your right knee as you straighten the right leg, and then start to lift your left knee as you straighten your left leg. Are you able to keep the same core engagement, tailbone tuck, and navel scoop as you did in a half plank? If not, you are not ready for any kind of plank. If you can and you feel comfortable exploring this, try peppering full planks in your practice, even for a second or two at a time.

Level 2: Roll Up

As you are doing your Diastasis Recti check, are you able to keep your tummy muscles in? Do you have that layer of support we mentioned in the check? Does it feel like you are in control of the movement around your entire core? Then pepper in very slow, controlled roll ups in your practice, just as many as you can do perfectly, and then stop. The rectus abdominis must be able to flex inward, never outward.

Level 3: Double Leg Lower/Lift

Lie on your back. Bring your knees into your chest. Support the back of your legs with your hands as you bring your knees over your hips. Let go with one hand. Is it in control? If not, stop here. If so, let go with the other hand. Is your back down, core engaged, navel scooped up? If so, start lowering your legs toward the ground. Stop wherever you cannot control, where your back starts to leave the floor, or where your navel starts losing ground. That's where to start with leg lowers and lifts. Don't push this exercise too fast or too soon. Gradually increase range.

Level 4: Pull-Down/Pull-Up

Hold an exercise band in both hands above your head. Stretch the band out to the sides as you make a half circle downward. Can you do this without opening the ribs? If so, continue. If not, stop there. Next, stand below a bar that you can hang from safely. Grab it start to lift one leg. If it feels wrong in your back or abdomen, stop immediately. If you are engaged and controlled, lift the other. Be very cautious here and take your time. If you can hang controlled, start to pull yourself up with your arms. This is the last stage in the exit protocol, so don't beat yourself up if this is impossible. You must be able to pull the navel up and in, and it should be pain free in order to progress into pull-ups and pull-downs. At any time, if it feels wrong, stop.

A word on leaving the group/high impact

We had mentioned previously that high impact exercise may not be a good choice at the time you are learning the methods in this book. At this point, if you are starting to feel strong through your midsection, see if you can leave the ground while pulling the navel up and in, and not losing posture and positioning. If that works for you, try a light jog. Err on the side of caution. If your organs are jostling or it feels like you're literally losing your guts, do not go back to impact just yet. You just need more muscle support first. Keep practicing the system and come back to this in a month, and just gauge your progress.

We are and always will be a work in progress. Do what you can do safely. Go to your boundaries but never past it. Work smarter, and stay safe. Your workouts may feel forever different because you are more in tune with what your muscles are actually doing. This will make every workout more effective, even if it is slower or in a different range of motion. Many people have never felt core engagement until going through this process, and than can start to feel like they are making headway in overall core health.

Overall core health leads to less pain, as well. The work you are doing here is for life. You can always come back to any of these sections to review elements of your personal strength. You will find that all of your overall strength comes from core connection and breath, and that is a very powerful discovery for life.

Chapter 10:

Consistency and Grace

Right about now, you may start to feel an overwhelming sense of not knowing.

"What's next?"

" How do I know?"

" What if I mess up?"

" How do I keep moving forward?"

" What if something gets in the way?" So, let's talk through some of these worries and hesitations.

Your keywords are **Consistency** and **Grace**. Be Consistent in your practice. Daily diligence in the ABC's and Life Lessons will be key to your healing. Being consistent in practicing the healing exercises in Chapter

9 will also help you strengthen and heal. If you lose consistency at any time, your best bet is just to come back to where you left off. Don't feel like you need to backtrack (except to review things you might have forgotten), but do not start completely OVER if you have just lost consistency along the way. You're just picking it back up and carrying it forward.

If you're carrying a loaf of bread home from the store and you drop it along the way, you may have to review where you have been, but you don't have to go back to making your grocery list and start completely over. You will go find where you left off and carry the bread home.

Have Grace for days that don't go as planned. Have Grace when you realize tomorrow what you didn't do today. You can only control today today, so stop worrying about what is past. Have Grace when you accidentally pick up something the wrong way. Just correct your form and move on. Have Grace when you feel something that feels off in your core. You may slap your forehead and say "Oh NO! I did something wrong!" Figure out what it is so that you can avoid it again, but don't beat yourself up for the next week because it happened. Pick up and move forward.

Who is in your life supporting you right now? A spouse? A friend? A family member? Even an older child? Tell that person what you are doing and why. Here is a script you can use if you don't know what to say.

"I have an injury. My stomach muscle opened while I was pregnant, and it is affecting my life. If I don't do anything about it, it could get worse. This opening causes me a lot of pain and discomfort. So, I found a system that can help me. This system requires that I do things differently for now. You might notice that I'm carrying fewer things around or that I am moving and doing things differently. It's all because I want this injury to heal for my health. Will you support me in this?"

Does all of this really MATTER? Well, yes it does. This healing process matters so much that your mind and body will thank you profusely when you start feeling better. Sometimes, the feeling better sounds like "oh…. That's different." Sometimes, it feels like "That doesn't kill my back anymore!" and sometimes, it feels like "Hm. That's different..." In other words, sometimes, the relief is over a period of time.

Your pictures should change over time. You may first notice an improved posture. You may feel you look taller or leaner. And then, you may notice flattening of the abdomen. Take pictures often. Stop being afraid of the camera like I used to be and take pictures to keep for yourself at least once a week. If you can, keep them in a folder or file, so that you can watch your progression.

You may be asking yourself, or me, at this point "How long is this going to take?" I wish I had a direct chart and I wish everything was as linear as "if this, then that." It's not that simple. I collect data as I go, with no direct line for healing time. Some people have seemingly large injuries and heal completely in the first six weeks. Some people seem to have a tiny injury that they are battling months down the road.

Here are some considerations to make, however. The number one indicator of healing over time seems to be

consistently following the ABC's. People who start and
continue the ABC's with intention tend to heal faster.
People who eat healthy and clean foods tend to heal
faster. This may be because of the ingredients we talked
about in Chapter 8. I like to think that is true. I don't
doubt the science of the power of food.
I do not notice any healing or recover correlation with
age, physical strength, height, or weight.

If you have discovered that you have a hernia, the
muscles may have a hard time closing over the hernia.
Most hernias interrupt the muscle healing just in that
one place. The good news is that you can close your
muscles around the hernia. The bad news is that you
can not exercise out a hernia, at least not in my practice.
Dr. Alina Sholar, Board Certified Plastic Surgeon in
Austin, Texas says "Do everything Carrie tells you.
Close the muscles around the hernia first, and then the
hernia repair is a small, outpatient surgery."

If you and your doctor decide to repair just the hernia, it
will be a simple practice of removing just that section.
He or she may not be concerned about the hernia, but if

it is hindering your life or if it is painful, consider having it removed. Recovery from a hernia surgery may take a couple of weeks. It is not the same as a full abdominoplasty (discussed in chapter 2).

Suppose things just don't seem to be going your way. You have been doing your very best to adhere to all of the guidelines in this book, and weeks or months later, you do not see any difference in your injury. What I usually see in this circumstance is an alignment problem. We usually have to schedule an alignment appointment to find exactly the point that is off for them. Contact me for help with alignment (tinyurl.com/carriefitscheduler or email carrie@carriefit.com) .

Another issue to your healing is intra-abdominal pressure, sometimes caused by visceral fat, and sometimes caused by internal swelling. Visceral fat collects around the internal abdominal organs and is the most dangerous form of fat in the body. This fat is pushing against the abdominal walls. If you have a protruding abdomen but can feel the muscles on the outside and soft tissue underneath, it may be visceral fat. Losing this weight will be critical to your healing and your overall health.

Finally, there are several foods that can cause abdominal swelling. This kind of swelling is also in the organs and digestive tract, which can swell and push against the muscles. Ask your local naturopath for help finding out if there is a food that is not agreeing with you. Some common food inflammatories are dairy, gluten, and soy.

One final block to address is your mental and spiritual health. In a recent study by the Ohio State University School of Psychiatry and Psychology, psychological stress can negatively affect the healing process. Consider having some kind of mental or spiritual practice that helps relieve some of the stress and pressure you may be feeling. In other studies, a 10 minute walk outside has the effect of reducing stress. Eating well and moving help reduce stress, as do a meditation practice or spiritual practices. Use the meditative practice in chapter 7 if it helps you. Seek guidance from a local spiritual leader or put a meditation practice in your schedule. Brainspace and Calm are popular meditation apps for iPhone. Alexa by Amazon also has meditation apps. Just a couple of minutes can change your mode from blocked to open. Stay open. Listen to the cues from your body. You will get through this.

Overall, we want you to be the healthiest version of yourself. Remember that taking care of any of these issues is not selfish. It is humble and selfless to take the time and energy you need to heal. You cannot pour from an empty cup.

Chapter 11:

She Who Went First

This method has gone from my self-therapy to a grand experiment to a skeleton of a method to a real system that really works. Some people have started this method with me from the time they accidentally met me somewhere. Some people searched me out from across the world.

When that initial PDF went viral and was shared throughout the world, I suddenly started receiving emails from Indonesia, Australia, Russia, and India, with pictures and testimonials that let me know for sure that I was on to something. The course that is now in this book has changed lives, not just bodies, and I am thrilled to be a piece of the puzzle for so many people.

I want to share these real stories with you because I know that some days you may not see the progress you want to see. Some days, you will want to give up. Some days, it will be hard. Some days, you will want to make an excuse. But if you will live by your magic words, Consistency and Grace, Life opens up.

Here are some words from some friends I have met along the way.

"I noticed no back pain for the past 2 days, and I feel like I'm standing taller because of changing my posture throughout the day. Plus I'm starting to notice that I'm not having to think about doing it. I am beginning to just do it throughout my day without thinking about it "- Krystle

"This program really does work!! I used it and closed my gap over an inch! Tested out of the program and now I'm doing two workouts a day! Guess what!! My gap is almost completely closed and my belly button is back to normal!!" - Kristin

"With Carrie's program combined with her fitness program support, I was able to get my gap down from 3-4 fingers wide to 0 to 1 finger wide, and I can do a lot of things I could not do before. No surgery, nothing drastic or expensive. I'd highly recommend her program." - Taylor

"My diastasis closed from 4.5 fingers to 2 fingers just from following the ABCs and your exercise modification suggestions *during pregnancy*! I'm so excited about that!" -Jatai

"My diastasis recti is almost completely healed! Which means if I continue to just not overdo ab work, and continue to strengthen my core, I can go back to full, unmodified workouts soon! Goodbye momma tummy!!!" - Bobbi

"Thank you Carrie. I am loving your program. You explain things very well. I feel my core is becoming stronger. This will only help with the healing that much more when I am finished nursing. I plan to continue the program over and over to keep a strong core and to remind myself to engage properly. One of my favourite things to do pre-pregnancy was sit-ups and work on my core. It wasn't until I had DR that I realized that I was doing it ALL wrong!" - Kerry

"I am also 2 years postpartum with my second baby. I have tried all sorts, other programmes, regular exercise, etc. and this is the first thing that's made any difference to my DR, and quickly too. I couldn't recommend it enough, even years postpartum" -Rachel

"Hi Carrie! Things have been going pretty good with my diastasis! I have seen a big improvement and lost some weight as well! I feel like I have caving in at my belly button more than I did before but maybe that is from the weight loss." -Kari

"I had Diastasis Recti, 4 fingers, and my connective tissue was completely destroyed. I would lay on the ground and my abs would bulge and my organs would spill out of my gap. It was uncomfortable beyond words. I was in rough shape. And I was a fitness instructor...... I kept thinking to myself, how in the world was I going to get into shape to teach again? How was I going to teach other people about fitness and health when my body looks like this? I was HARD on myself. I started researching diastasis recti and trying different exercises. Carrie's was the first program I completed and it helped me SO MUCH.My core is stronger then ever AND I still have a gap! But I keep up on my exercises and BREATHING ". -Meg

"Very helpful in gradually increasing core strength even if the core is very weak or has significant injury. Saw improvement quickly with a small amount of daily time commitment which makes it great for moms who are recovering after a birth or who have small children." - Rebecca

"I just took my measurements after finishing my second round of the Diastasis Recti Recovery System. When I started, my DR was approximately 1.25" wide, 1" deep, and 4" long. Today, it is approximately 1" wide, 1/2" deep, and 1.5" long. It's definitely a process, but it's working! "- Leslie

"Carrie is the First instructor to ever address the day to day limitations I have with my DR core injury and to explain that the abdomen muscles can flex in as well as push out! GREAT setup for my participation in the rest of the course- because, after all, what good is doing 6 weeks of therapy work if I'm just "undoing" all that work with my daily bad posture?" - Meredith

"First and foremost I want to thank you so much for all you do to help those of us with Diastasis Recti! Your modification videos for the 21 Day fix program (and other programs!) have been so valuable I can't even tell you! As I mentioned in a previous email it's given me a joy back that I thought I lost! Being able to workout without fear of making my injury worse! "- Courtney

"Yes! And honestly I feel like the modifications in itself has helped so much too, because I am working on core strength without doing more damage! I did more damage over the last year when I didn't know I had DR and kept doing everything I'm not really supposed to. The combination of modifying and your program will do the trick and then I'll have to deal w my hernia. But one thing at a time!" Claudia

"I just started the DR program and have an umbilical hernia! After day one I'm already seeing my belly shrink!!!" - Stacey

"By cracking down on it, I am CLOSING MY GAP. Seriously. Now, I'm about 1.5 above the navel, 1 finger below the navel, and (this was the kicker) LESS than ONE finger wide. Like I have to turn my finger sideways now to measure.
I'm not stopping there, except maybe for a leap of excitement and celebration! Once I get this closed, I can work on restrengthening the full core so I can have a flat stomach for the first time in over 13 years.

Thank you for all of your awesome support, Carrie!!!" -
Gina

"I LOVE you. So thankful you don't keep this to yourself
because it has changed my life."
- Sonja

Every client is different. Every body is different. Every
life is different. Every injury is different. Every journey is
different. Here is what has remained the same: Healing
Happens with Consistency and Grace. You can do this,
even on the days it seems hard. And on the days it
seems hardest, you're going to lean on your support
system. You're going to ask for help. But you are not
going to resign yourself to lose out on life, to live in pain,
or to consider yourself unworthy of healing. Your body
and your mind are worth everything. This is your life,
and I want you to live it and Love It.

Acknowledgements

I would like to acknowledge those in the pre and post natal field, who strive every day to make pre and postnatal care better for women and babies. There are thousands of midwives, doulas, doctors, therapists, and specialists who believe in better care for mothers worldwide, and put in their long and difficult hours every day to teach mothers and families about self care and care practices.

I would like to acknowledge all of my Pilates and yoga teachers, as well as several people in chiropractic care, who have taught me what the body is capable of. I would like to especially acknowledge **Dr. Melissa Vrazel**, a chiropractor in Texas, for teaching me about alignment and helping me find my own for the first time. I would like to acknowledge **Tandy Gutierrez**, who helped me really understand the power of the Pilates method and what it really means when practiced correctly.

Thank you, Mothers of the World, for acknowledging that you deserve a healthy life free from pain, and thank you for paying that message forward.

About the Author

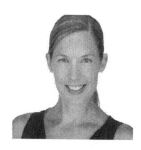

Carrie Harper is a fitness professional with over 20 years of experience in group and personal training. She is a writer, speaker, and teacher in all things fitness and a specialist in pre and post natal fitness. Carrie has spent the last 10 years studying and developing therapy systems to help post natal women recover from childbirth, particularly from the very common core injury, Diastasis Recti, left undiagnosed in most postnatal women.

Carrie had Diastasis Recti as a new mother in 2005, and was given no help or advice on the topic from the medical industry, or from her own industry, fitness. After a long, hard battle with injury, surgery, and surgery recovery, she became her own therapist, digging into her library of studies in the many fields of exercise and wellness. Much to her delight, when she started using the therapies on her own clients, they started to heal from Diastasis Recti.

In 2014, her first published technique, on a simple PDF labeled "The Flat Belly System" went worldwide and surprised Carrie at the widespread healing that was happening. From there, she developed a more complete system to help people from the initial finding of the injury through the process of healing, including an exit strategy and overall life lessons and adjustments. Through these programs, Carrie has been overwhelmed with letters of appreciation for her therapies and extra help.

Carrie lives in Austin, Texas, with husband Eric, and her two daughters.

Contact Information:

Carrie Harper:
Email: carrie@carriefit.com
Website: www.carriefit.com
Social Media:

www.facebook.com/carriefit

www.instagram.com/carriefit

www.youtube.com/user/carriefit

Free Diastasis Recti Special Help Group:

https://www.facebook.com/groups/carriefitdiastasisrecti/

Made in the USA
Middletown, DE
18 January 2020